FINDING REBECCA

The Forgotten Life of Dr. Rebecca Lee Crumpler,
America's First Black Female Doctor

Written by
Shani Mahiri King

Illustrated by
Nicole Tadgell

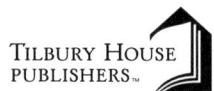

an imprint of
Cherry Lake Publishing Group
2395 South Huron Parkway, Suite 200
Ann Arbor, MI 48104
www.tilburyhouse.com

Printed and bound in South Korea

10 9 8 7 6 5 4 3 2 1

Library of Congress Cataloging-in-Publication Data

Names: King, Shani Mahiri, author. | Tadgell, Nicole, 1969- illustrator.
Title: Finding Rebecca : the forgotten life of Dr. Rebecca Lee Crumpler, America's
first Black female doctor / written by Shani Mahiri King ; illustrated by Nicole
Tadgell. Other titles: Forgotten life of Dr. Rebecca Lee Crumpler, America's first
Black female doctor Description: Ann Arbor : Tilbury House Publishers, 2024. |
Audience: Ages 7-12 | Summary: "This book examines the casual disappearance
of America's first Black female doctor from records and memory. But author
Shani King uses the few details we do have to piece together a picture of the life
she led, her hardships, and her many accomplishments" -- Provided by publisher.

Identifiers: LCCN 2024011328 | ISBN 9781958394083 (hardcover)
Subjects: LCSH: Crumpler, Rebecca Lee, 1831-1895. |
African American women physicians--Massachusetts--Boston--Biography. |
African American physicians--Massachusetts--Boston--Biography. |
African American physicians--United States--History--19th century. |
Women physicians--Massachusetts--Boston--Biography. |
Physicians--Massachusetts--Boston--Biography.
Classification: LCC R154.C852 K56 2024 | DDC 610.92 [B]--dc23/
eng/20240516 LC record available at https://lccn.loc.gov/2024011328

FINDING REBECCA

The Forgotten Life of Dr. Rebecca Lee Crumpler,
America's First Black Female Doctor

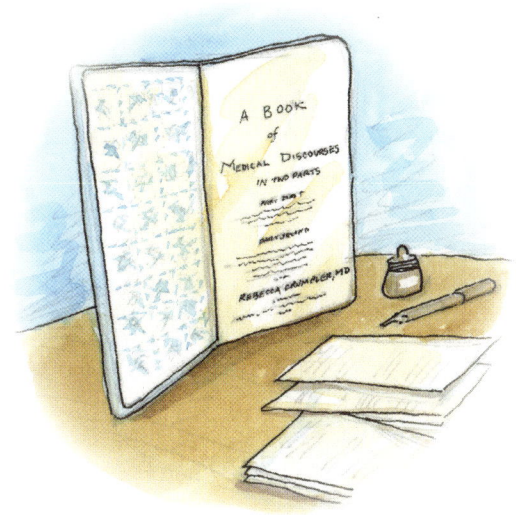

Written by
Shani Mahiri King

Illustrated by
Nicole Tadgell

TILBURY HOUSE PUBLISHERS

HER LIFE WAS A HERO'S JOURNEY.

HER ACHIEVEMENTS WERE
TRIUMPHS OVER ADVERSITY.

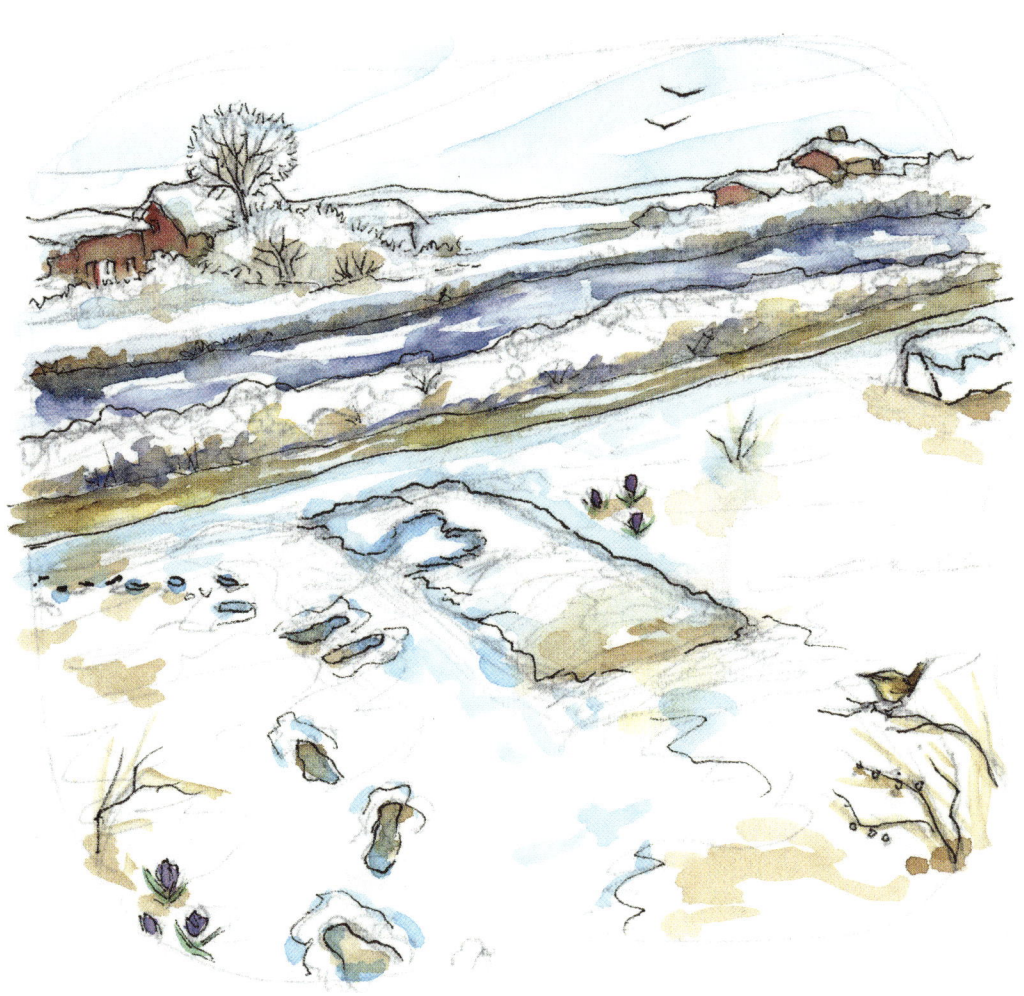

SHE WAS A TRAILBLAZER.
SHE **SHOULD** BE FAMOUS.
WHY HAVE WE NEVER HEARD OF HER?

The story of Rebecca Lee Crumpler begins with an unmarked grave.

Abandoned and anonymous, solitary and mysterious.

A mystery of history, you might say.

All memory of the first Black woman medical doctor in the United States seemingly vanished into her grave with her in 1895. She lay there forgotten in the Boston, Massachusetts, neighborhood of Hyde Park for 125 years.

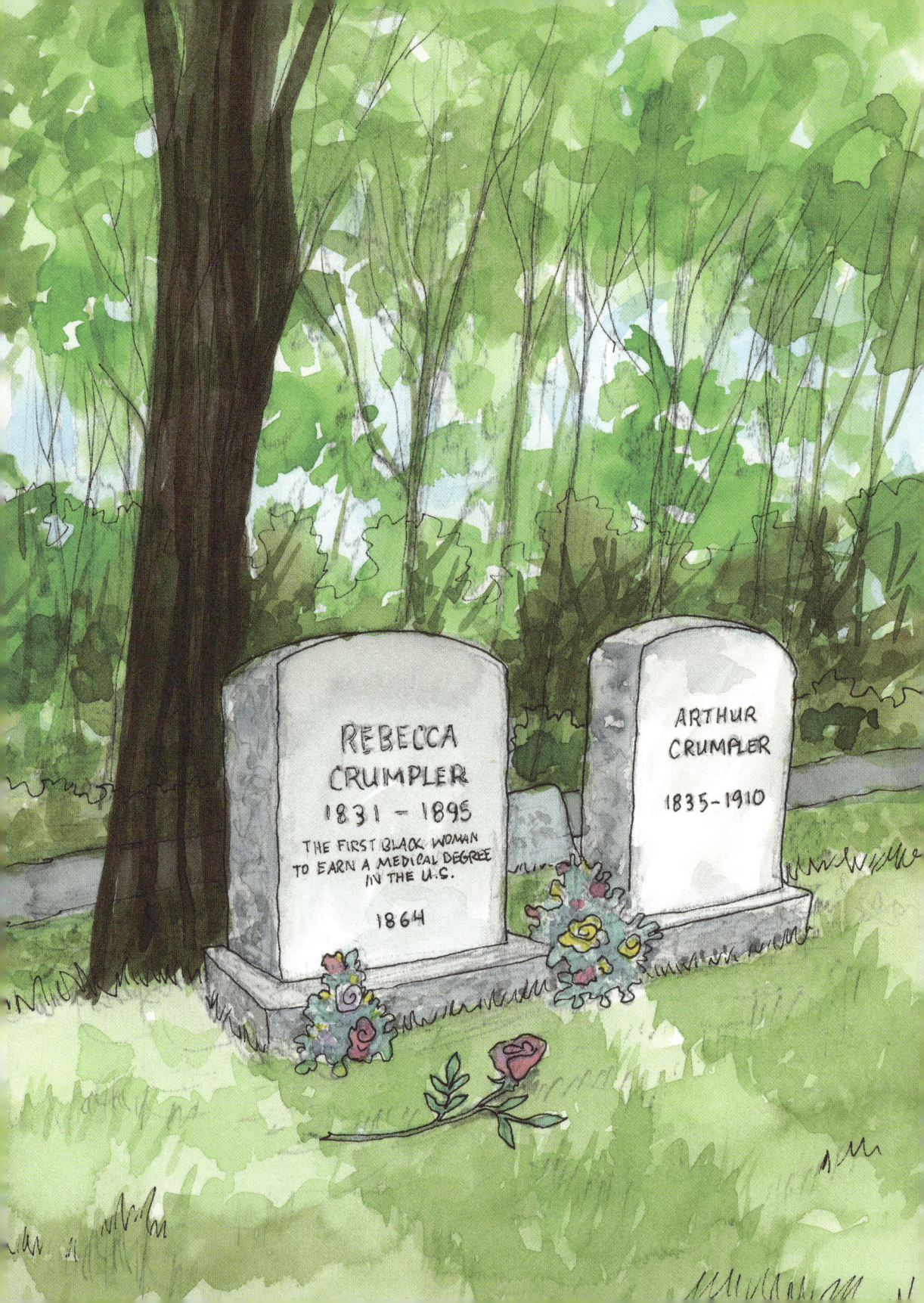

125 YEARS!!!

But a dedicated group of physicians at last succeeded in locating Rebecca's burial place, and in June 2020 she received a proper headstone. The following year, on the 190th anniversary of her birth, the city of Boston declared February 8th to be Dr. Rebecca Lee Crumpler Day.

You might think this is the end of the story, but really it is the beginning. Who was Rebecca? How did she become a doctor with the odds stacked against her? What obstacles did she have to overcome? What made her strong? Who helped her along the way?

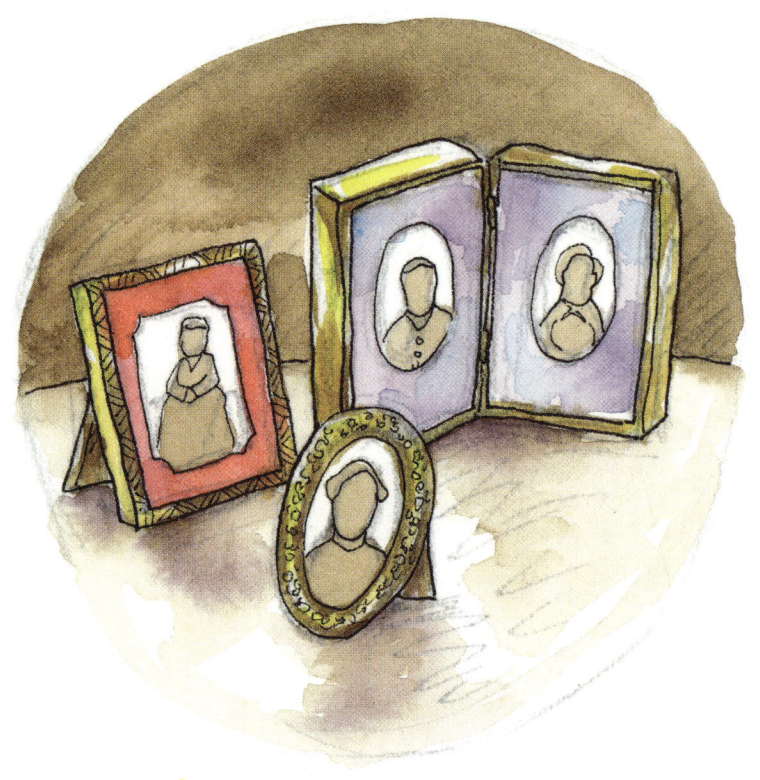

And why don't we know more about this amazing American?

There are very few sources of information available on Rebecca. She was described in her early sixties as being "tall and straight, with light brown skin and gray hair." More than that? Well, we don't know. Searches of libraries and online databases for books, journals, newspaper archives, censuses, and other historic records that might mention her name lead to one dead end after another.

Among the earliest photos of Black Americans are four daguerreotypes (early photographs that used silver plates instead of film) of enslaved people created before the Civil War, now in the collections of Harvard University. Photography was much more common after the war—by which time Rebecca was an accomplished doctor in her thirties—yet no verified images of her have been found. Were photos taken of her but later lost? Are they tucked away in a drawer somewhere, unlabeled, still awaiting discovery? Was she simply deemed unimportant enough to photograph, perhaps because she was a woman? What a contrast with Frederick Douglass, her fellow Black trailblazer, who died the same year and was the most photographed person of the nineteenth century!

Fortunately, there is one book that helps.

A book written by Rebecca herself.

In 1883, Rebecca Crumpler published a handbook titled *Medical Discourses*, which was one of the first medical publications by a Black American. In the front of the book, she dedicated it to:

> nurses, mothers and to all who may desire to
> mitigate the suffering of the human race.

In its introduction, Rebecca provided the only first-person narrative we have for her life. It is woefully incomplete—its purpose was to introduce a medical handbook, not to be an autobiography—but it provides a starting point for research into Rebecca's story.

She was born in 1831 in the small town of Christiana, Delaware. Her birth name was Rebecca Davis, and her parents were Absalom and Matilda Webber Davis.

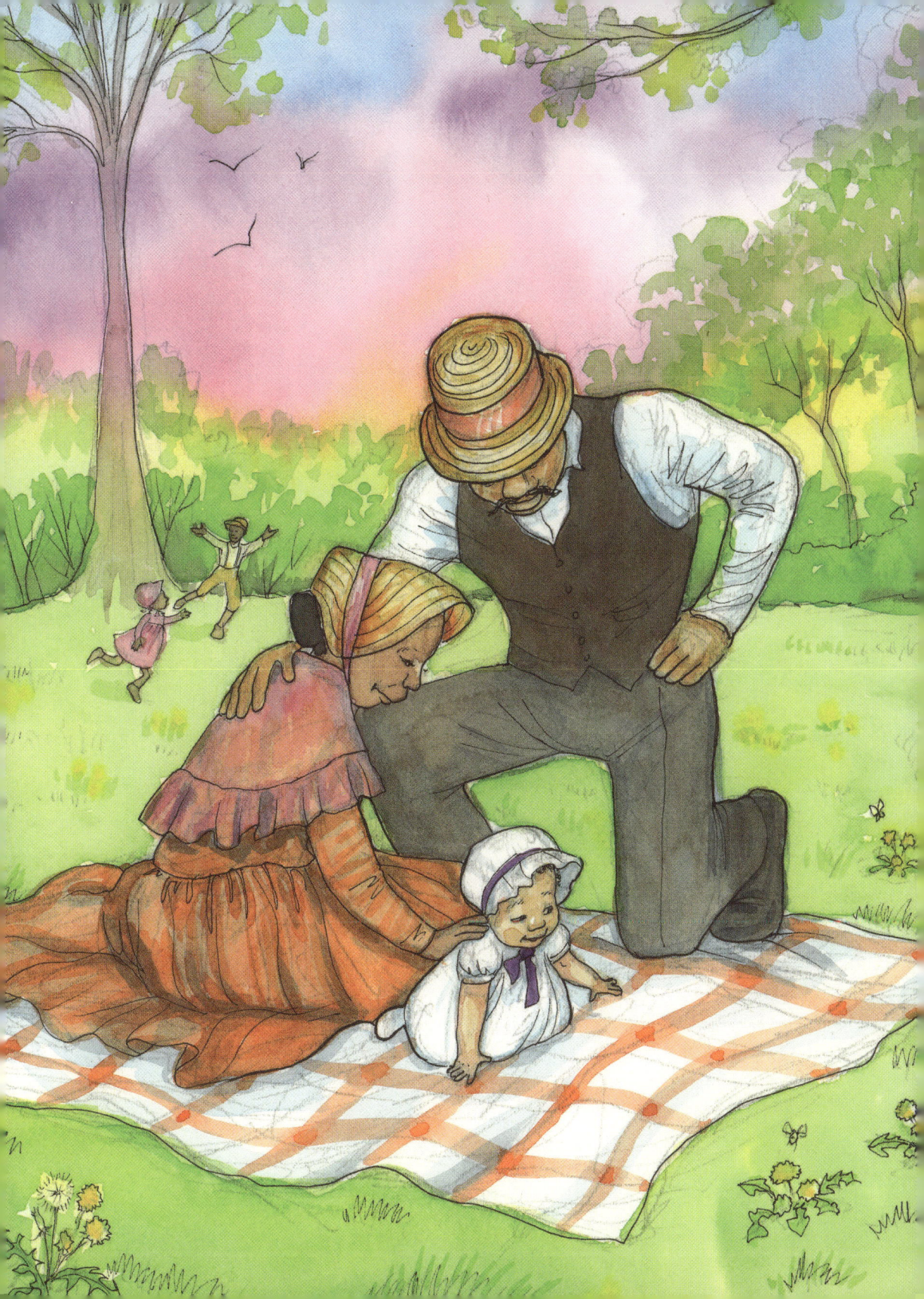

Most Black people in America were enslaved back then, but Rebecca was born free—as were many Black residents of Delaware. Christiana is close to Wilmington, DE, a major city offering more work opportunities for Black people than many other places at the time. In Wilmington, Black men and women owned businesses and were skilled tradespeople—tanners, blacksmiths, grocers, and barbers. Jobs were more limited outside the city, where Black folks were often farmworkers or domestic laborers. Because farms in Delaware were generally much smaller than in the Southern states, farmers found it cheaper to hire Black laborers than to buy slaves, and this too promoted the freedmen's culture in Delaware. Free and enslaved Black laborers were instrumental in the building of critical public works projects like the Chesapeake and Delaware Canal.

By 1810, Delaware had a larger proportion of free people in its African American population (76 percent) than New York (63 percent) or New Jersey (42 percent). By 1840, Delaware had the largest free Black population (by percentage of population) in America. Delaware's communities were heavily influenced by the Society of Friends—the Quakers—who promoted equality, shared work, and education. The Quakers, known for their faith in the equality of all people and their opposition to social injustices, believed that the education of freedmen would improve not just Black citizens but society as a whole—an uncommon idea at the time.

We know little about Rebecca's early life. Her family left no records—at least none that have been found—and Black people were not much written about in white-owned newspapers of the time, especially women and girls. *Our National Progress,* the first Black-owned newspaper in Delaware, wouldn't appear until 1869, three decades after Rebecca left Christiana.

When Rebecca was a girl, there was no guarantee of public schooling. Although some states did offer a small number of schools, kids were often excluded on the basis of race, income, gender, and geography.

A few schools that would enroll Black children were eventually established in Delaware with funds from Black landowners, the Quakers, and the Methodist Episcopal Church, but this probably happened too late to benefit Rebecca. Like many other African American children of the time, she was likely educated by family and friends.

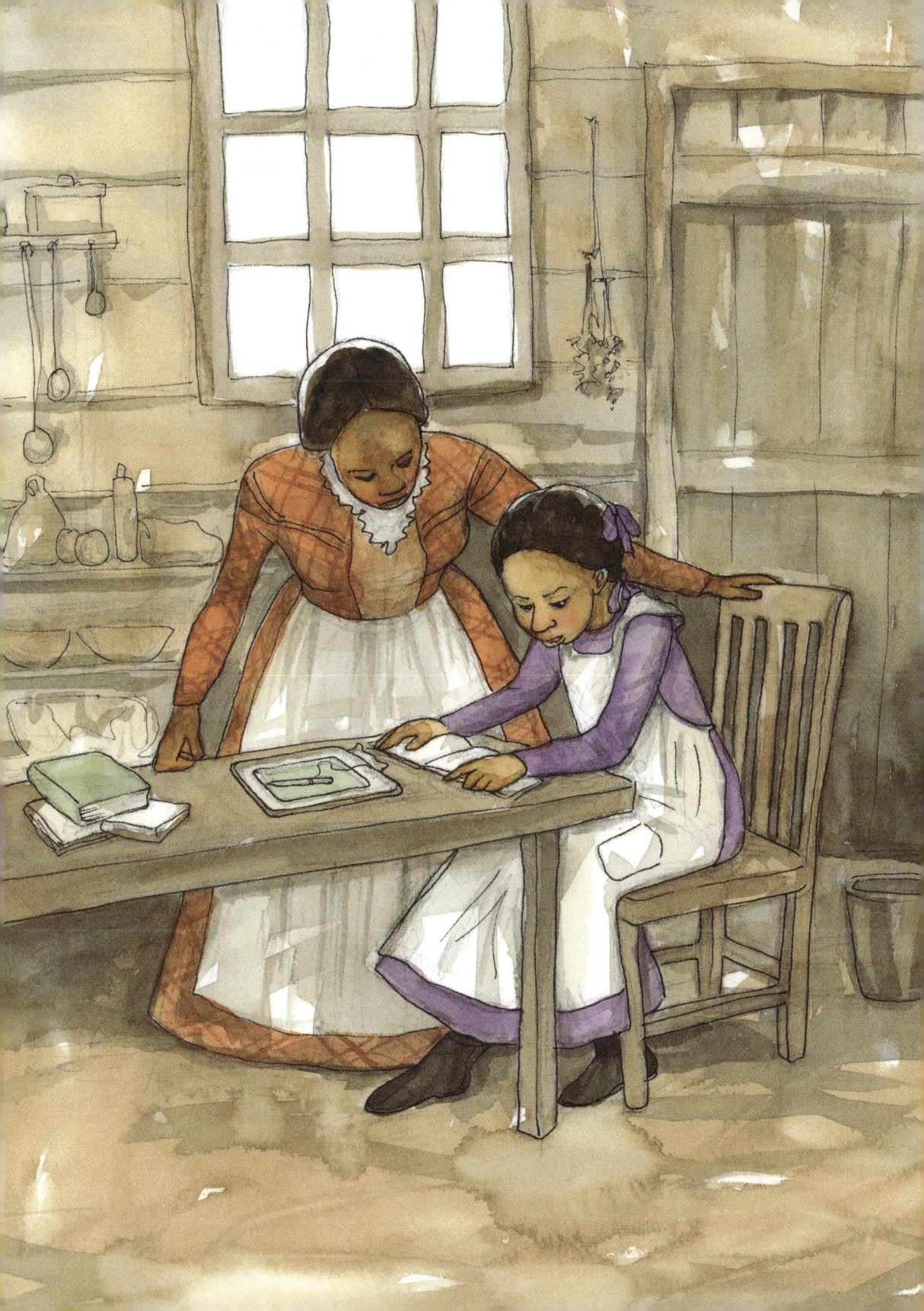

At a young age, Rebecca went to live with an aunt, Eliza Davis, in Philadelphia, Pennsylvania. We don't know how old she was at the time, but she must have been very young, because Rebecca would write in the introduction to her book that her aunt had raised her.

A new railroad connecting Wilmington and Philadelphia was completed in 1836, and Rebecca may have ridden the train north to meet her aunt. The journey was only thirty miles but, for Black people, travel required bravery and determination.

Did she make the trip alone? It seems more likely that an adult traveled with her. Perhaps her father left his young daughter with his sister in Philadelphia and then made a sad and fearful journey home. We don't know.

After the slave rebellion led by Nat Turner in 1831, laws were passed in many states limiting the rights of slaves to travel, gather, or be educated. Any Black person wishing to travel needed an official note, called an affidavit, signed by a white citizen. Such affidavits were rarely sought and even more rarely granted, which essentially made travel illegal for Black Americans.

To make matters worse, Delaware was a border state between the free Northern states and the slaveholding South. Escaped slaves often passed through border states on their harrowing journeys north. Frederick Douglass is said to have escaped slavery in Maryland aboard a Philadelphia, Wilmington & Baltimore train. Federal law at the time permitted Southern slaveholders to pursue and capture their escaped "property" in the North, which meant that Black folks traveling in Delaware were in danger of being captured by bounty hunters or corrupt police officers even if they had never been enslaved. It was common for free African Americans to be detained and "returned" to the South into slavery.

There must have been a reason for Rebecca's family to send her away so young. Maybe one or both of her parents had died, as happened often in that time of cholera, tuberculosis, and other epidemics. Perhaps Rebecca showed an early interest in medicine. Perhaps her family wanted an education for her that could not be had in Delaware.

But we do know that Rebecca developed great affection for the aunt who played such a large role in her life.

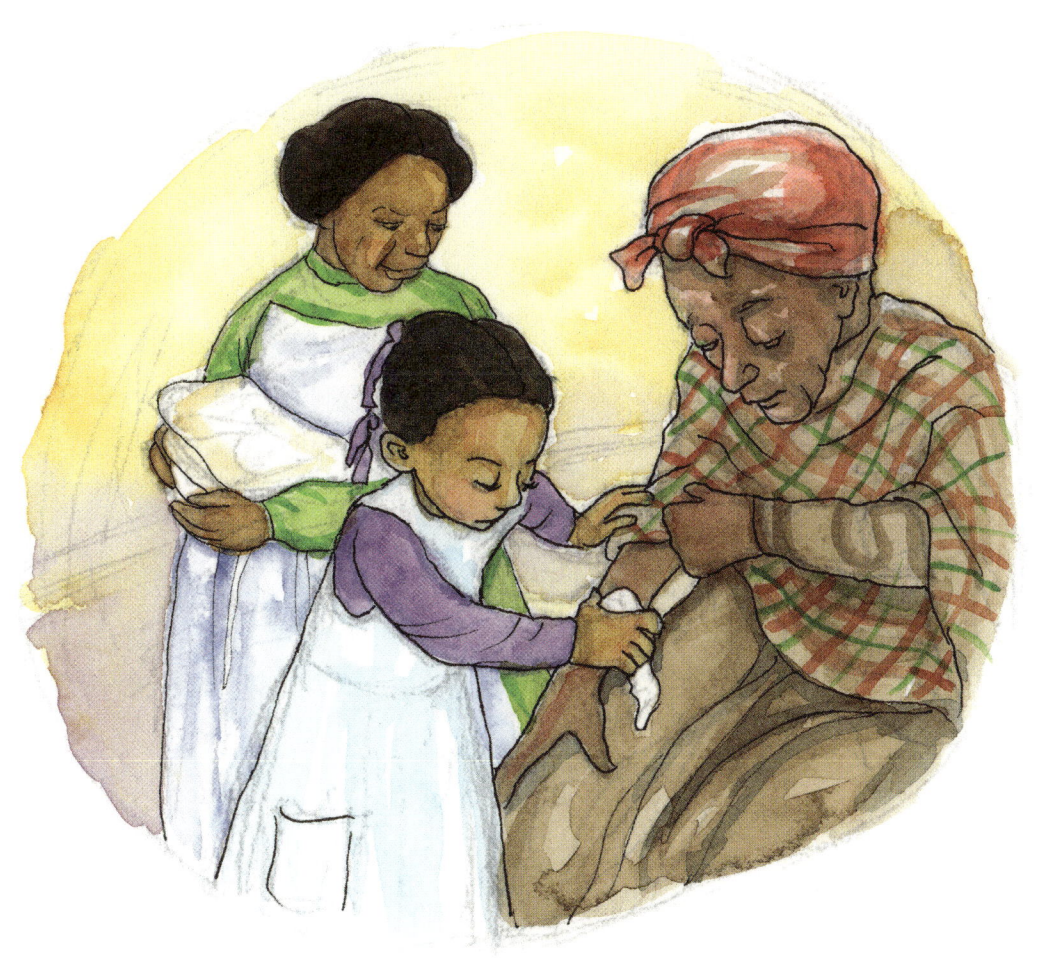

"Having been reared by a kind aunt whose usefulness with the sick was continually sought . . . I early conceived a liking for and sought every opportunity to be in a position to relieve the suffering of others."

—DR. REBECCA LEE CRUMPLER

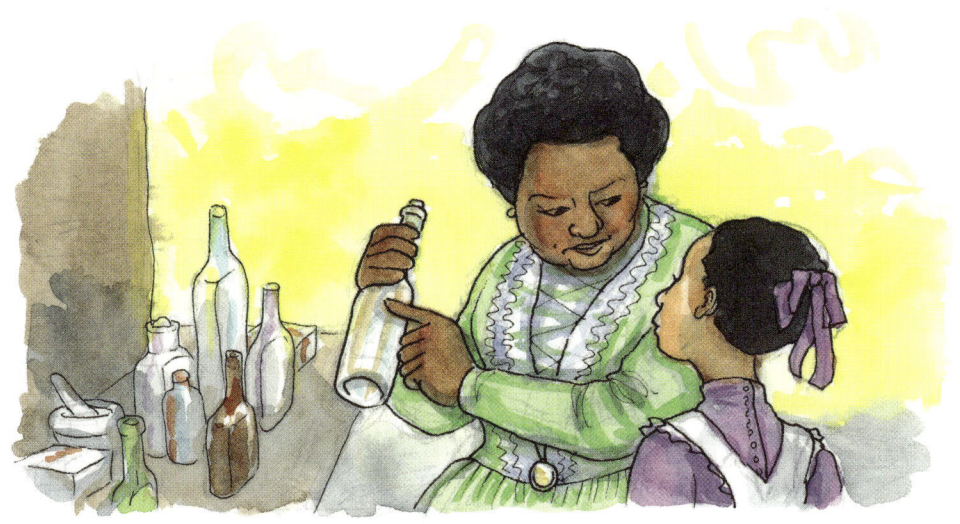

According to an 1850 city directory, they lived at 117 Christian Street, an address that no longer exists. We know that Aunt Eliza Davis was born around 1810, but we don't know whether she ever married or had children of her own.

We know from Rebecca's own words that Eliza was a caring woman, a community health worker beloved by those she served. Eliza likely had not gone to nursing school, but probably had learned from a network of Black women caregivers and midwives. Most Black midwives, both free and enslaved women, learned traditional healing arts and practices that were passed down through families or in apprenticeships.

"This may have been where I developed my love for caregiving, one of the many things for which I became known."

—DR. REBECCA LEE CRUMPLER

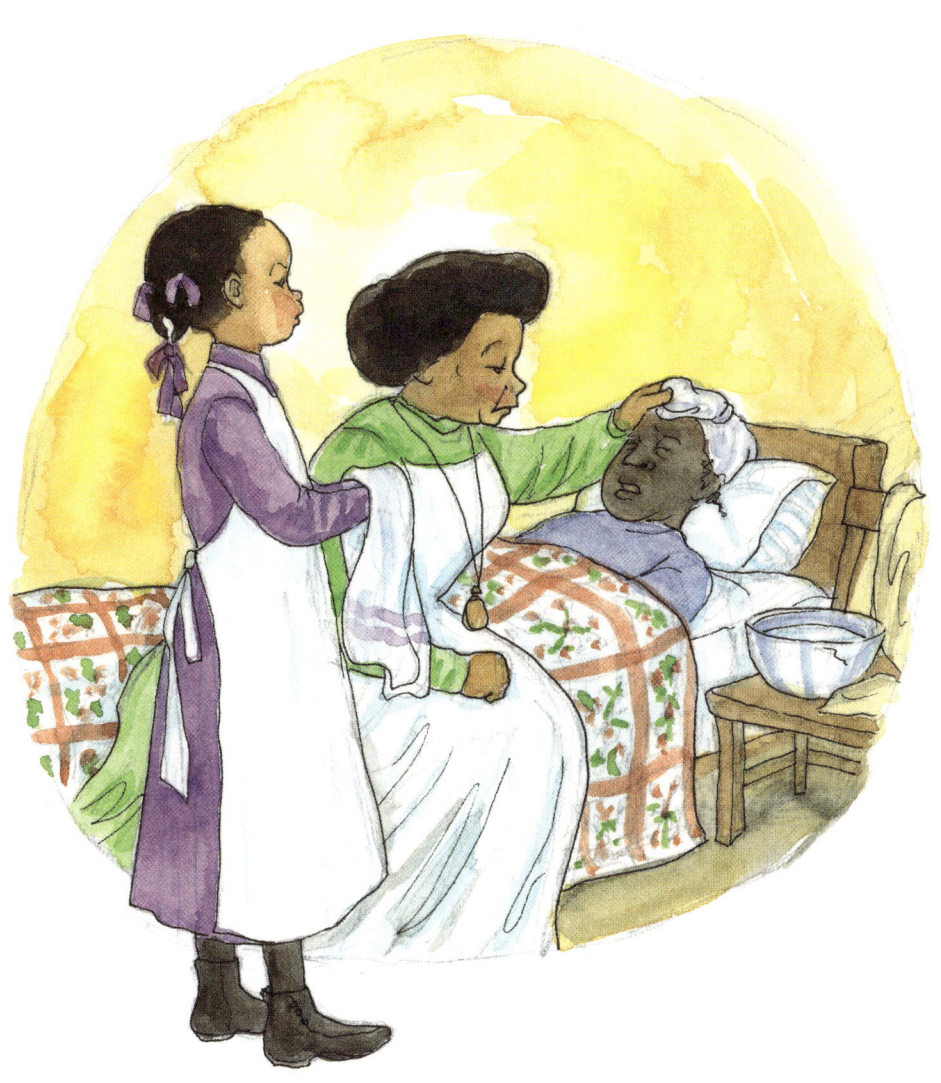

Rebecca seems to have lived with her aunt for a decade or more. And then, at the age of seventeen, Rebecca traveled north again—this time all the way to the West Newton English and Classical School outside Boston, Massachusetts. The school embraced a diverse student population and enrolled students across age, race, and gender.

All students took sports, dancing, singing, music, painting, drawing, geography, writing, physical science, classical literature, astronomy, public speaking, bookkeeping, and mathematics. In addition to skilled, engaged, well-paid teachers, students enjoyed drop-in lectures from artists, intellectuals, and politicians.

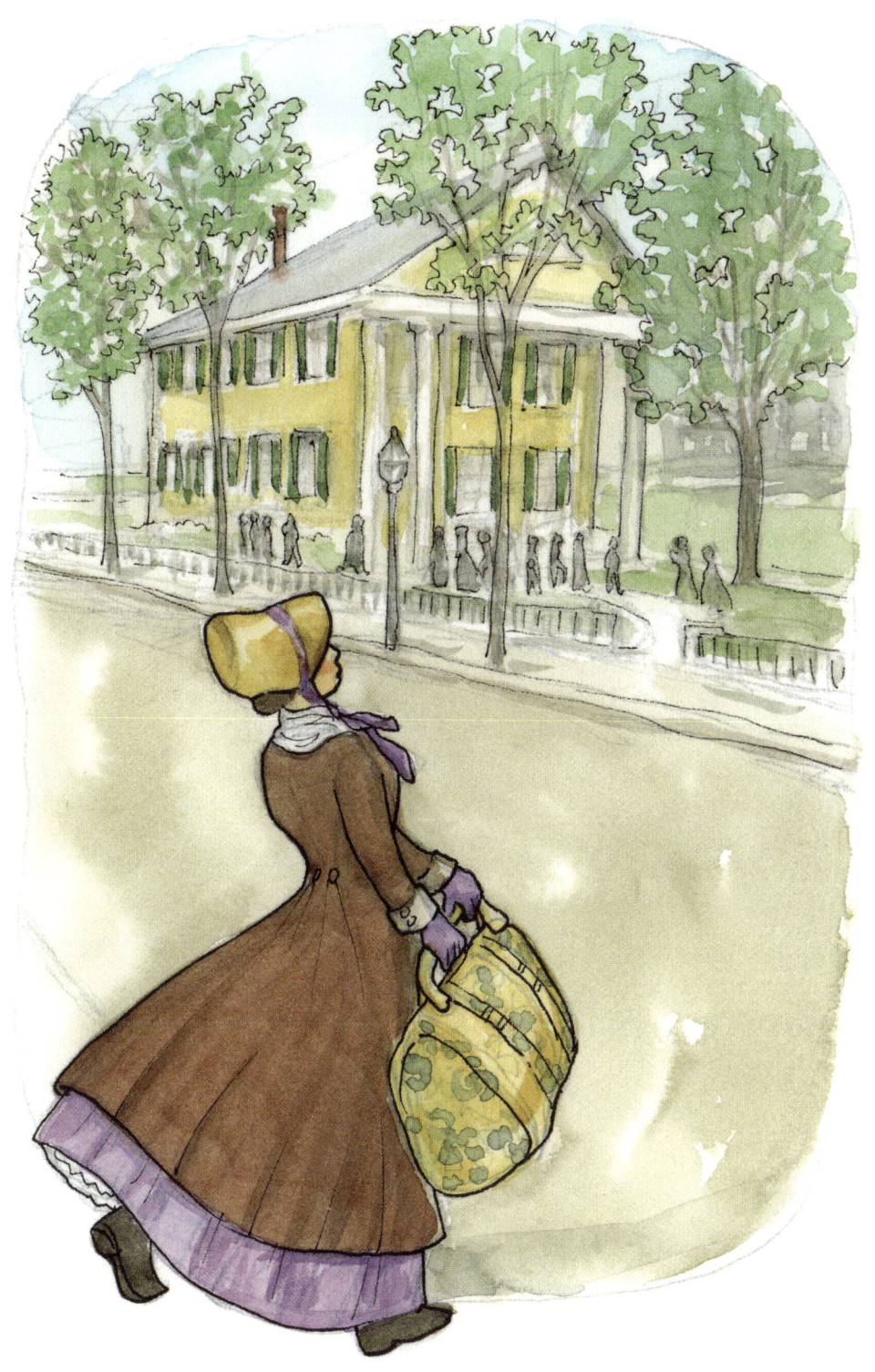

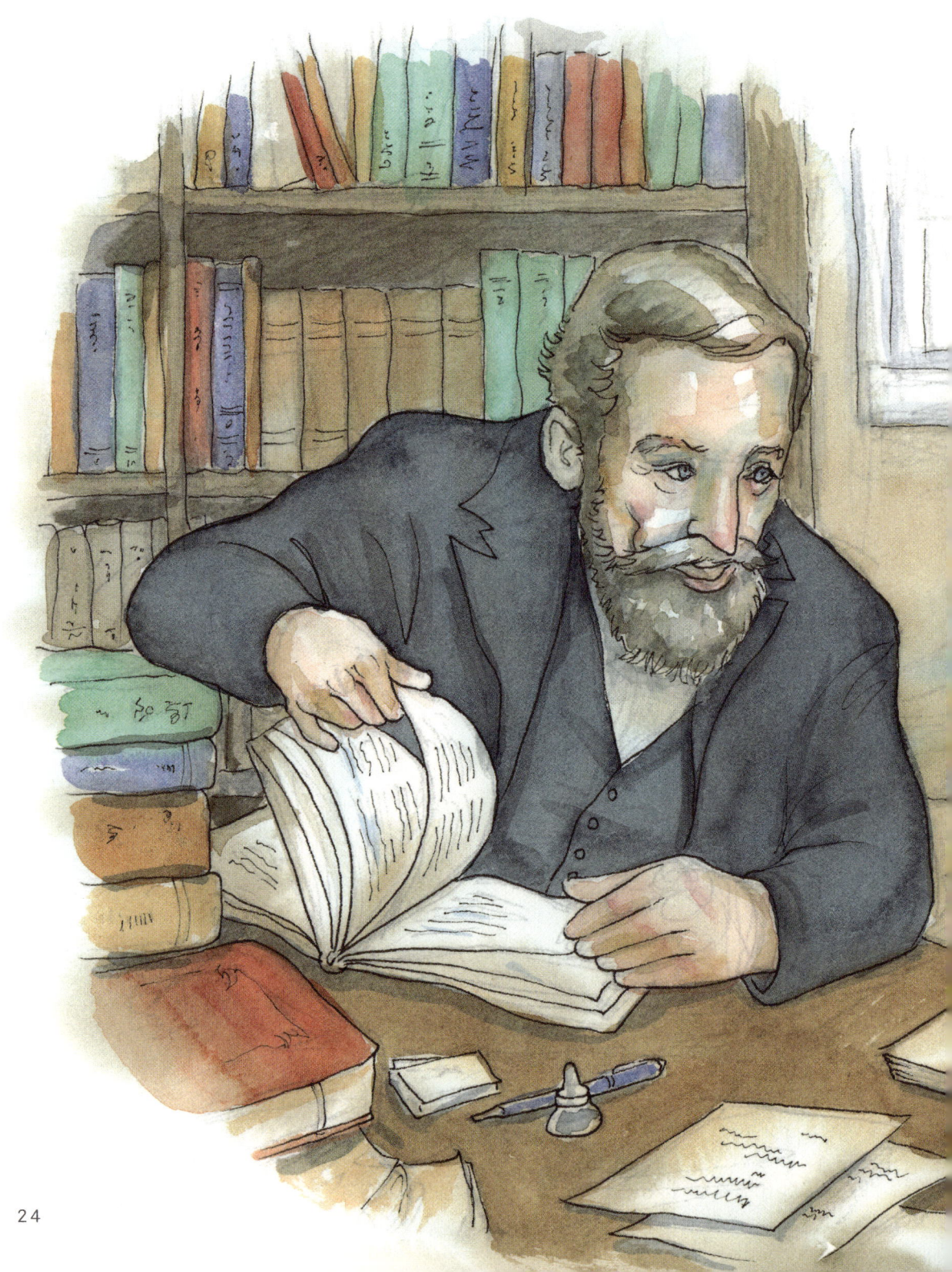

Rebecca's interest in medicine was nurtured in the natural science classes the school was known for. She worked hard, developing strong reading, writing, and mathematics skills. She took extra courses in math and studied directly with the president of the school, Nathaniel Allen.

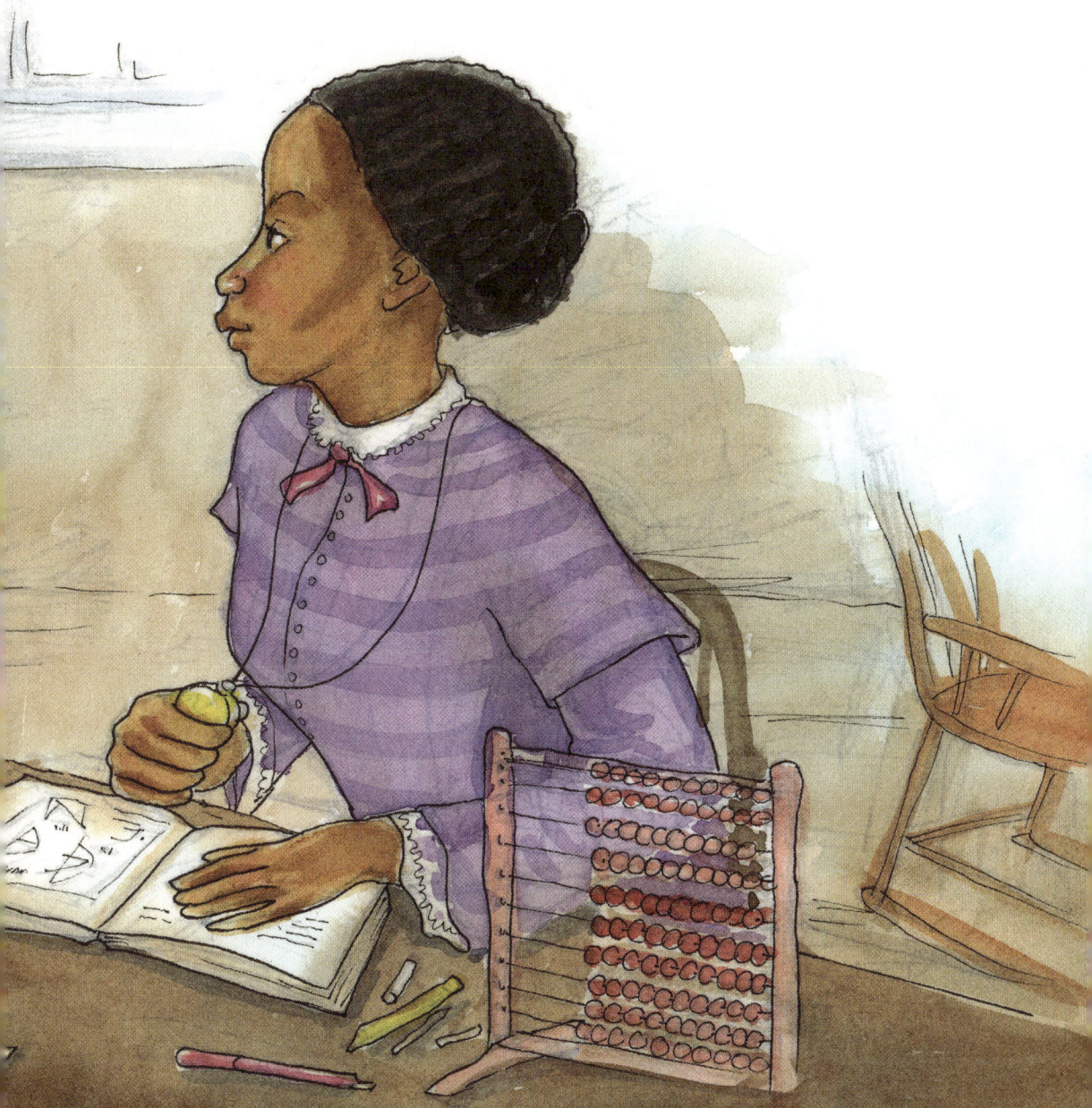

There were not many Black students at West Newton at the time, and Rebecca was one of the oldest students there, most being fifteen or younger. How did she get this opportunity? How did she make the journey from Philadelphia to Boston? We don't know. We only know that she made the most of the chance she was given.

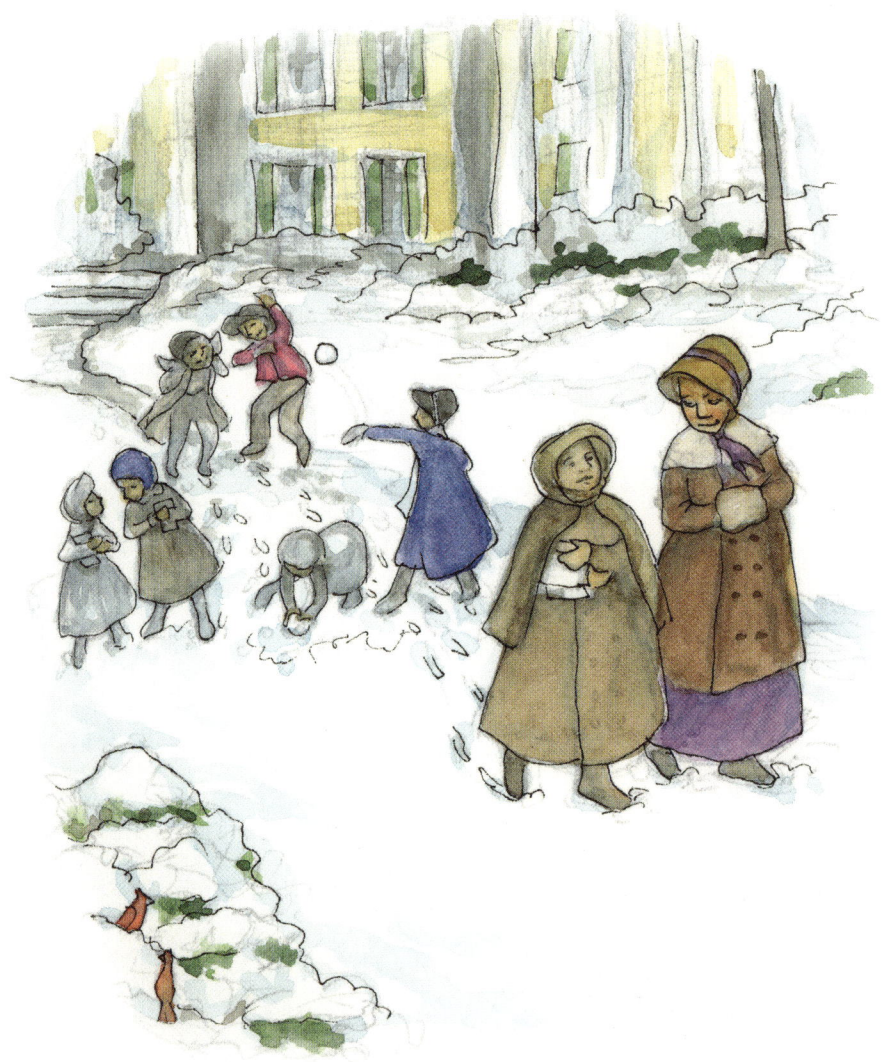

West Newton is today one of thirteen villages within the city of Newton, but in 1850 it was a small hamlet of 500 people ten miles west of Boston. The town was ruled by a conservative Orthodox Christian church that disapproved of Nathaniel Allen's modern educational vision for West Newton English and Classical School. The conservative community wanted narrow teachings focused on order and Christian lessons, but Allen persisted in offering recreation and creative subjects in order to educate the whole person.

He enrolled Black students and women from the beginning, reflecting his abolitionist and women's rights politics, even as surrounding schools that attempted to enroll Black students were attacked for doing so. Nathaniel's wife and an extended family of aunts, uncles, and cousins served as teachers and administrators. Many of the students stayed with Allen family members while attending the school.

Nathaniel Allen's school shows the impact even one good school can have on the lives of children.

In 1852, after four years of studies, Rebecca married Wyatt Lee, a formerly enslaved man. We don't know how they met, but Rebecca was well known in the Boston area's Black community. She moved from West Newton to Boston with Wyatt and worked both in her own practice and with doctors there as a nurse—and excelled in the field. Available historical materials suggest that Rebecca focused much of her personal training and practice on the care of mothers and young children.

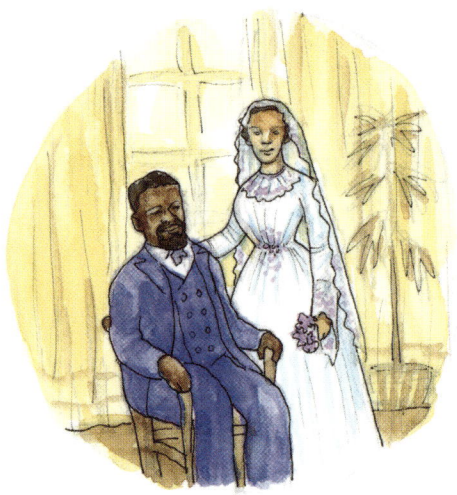

Most medical work was done in patients' homes at the time, so Rebecca likely traveled in and around Boston, which helped her build strong roots in the community. Very few Black women were doing what she was doing. Very few had been granted the opportunity.

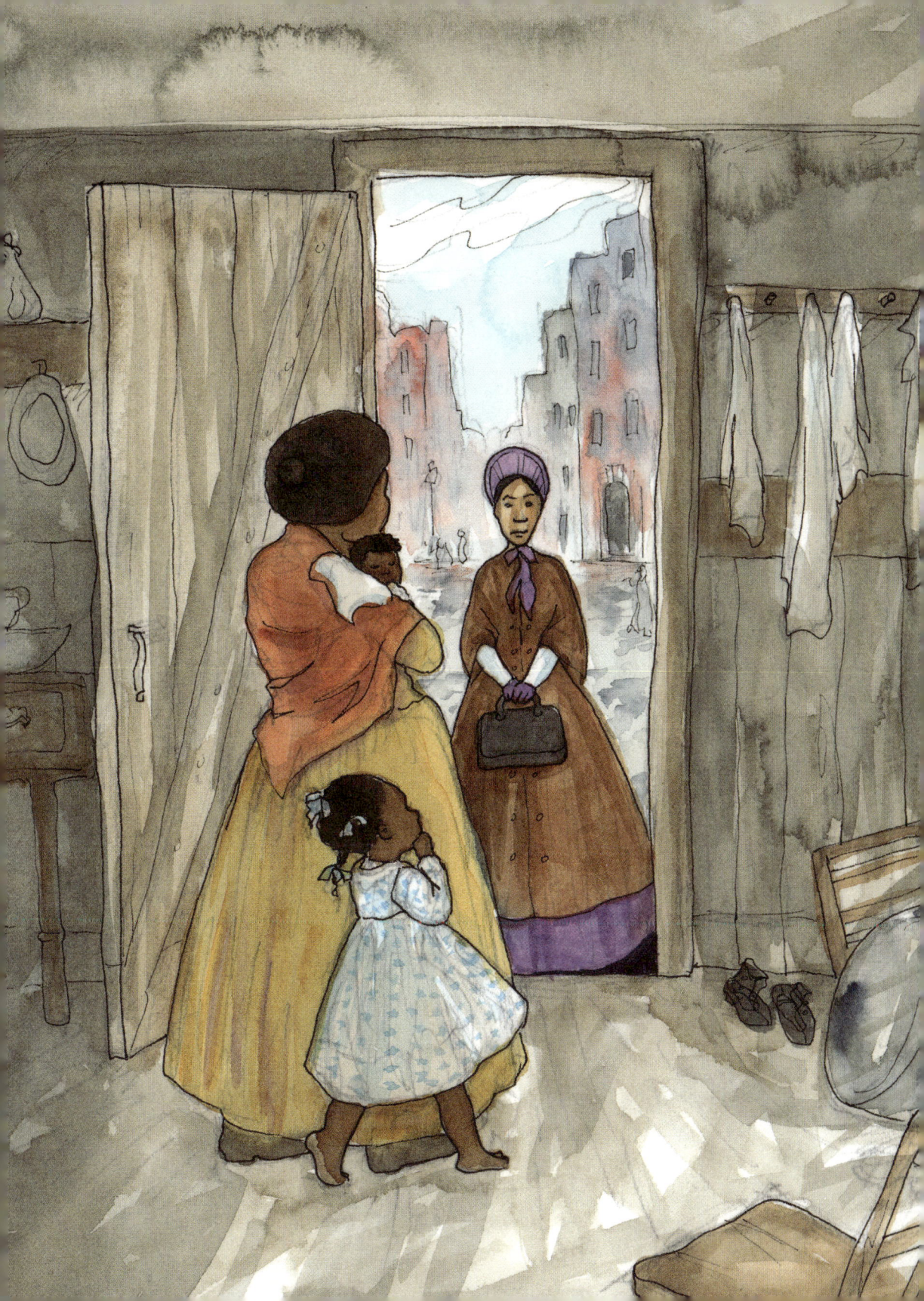

Because she excelled, she received letters of commendation from the doctors she worked with, which was even more unusual for a Black woman of the time. Then, in 1860, she applied and was admitted to the New England Female Medical College, where she became the first Black student.

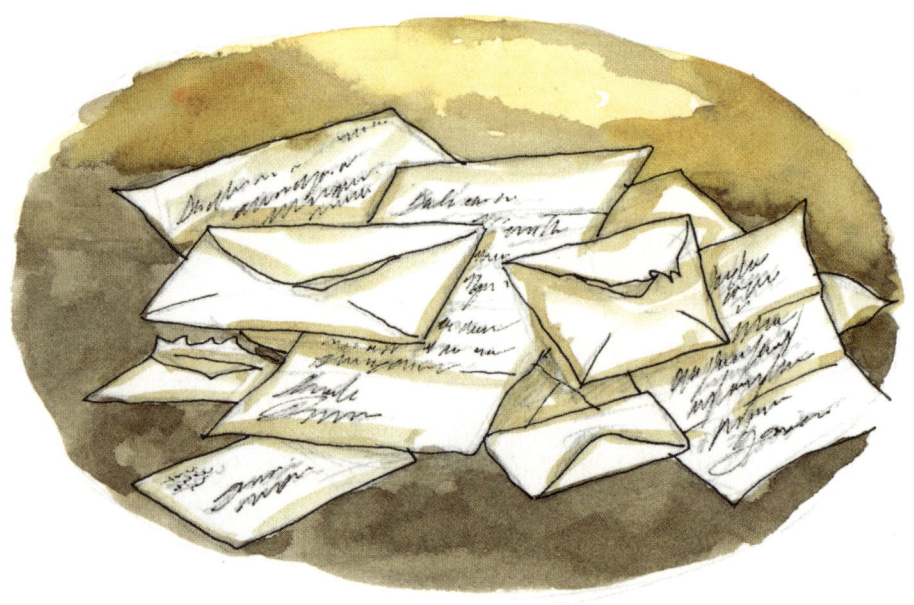

"From these doctors I received letters commending me to the faculty of the New England Female Medical College."

—DR. REBECCA LEE CRUMPLER

Rebecca studied there as much as she could over the next four years. It was a hard time. The Civil War began in the spring of 1861, and money was tight. The school suspended courses so that students and faculty could help care for wounded Union soldiers. Rebecca also had to care for Wyatt, who died of tuberculosis in 1863.

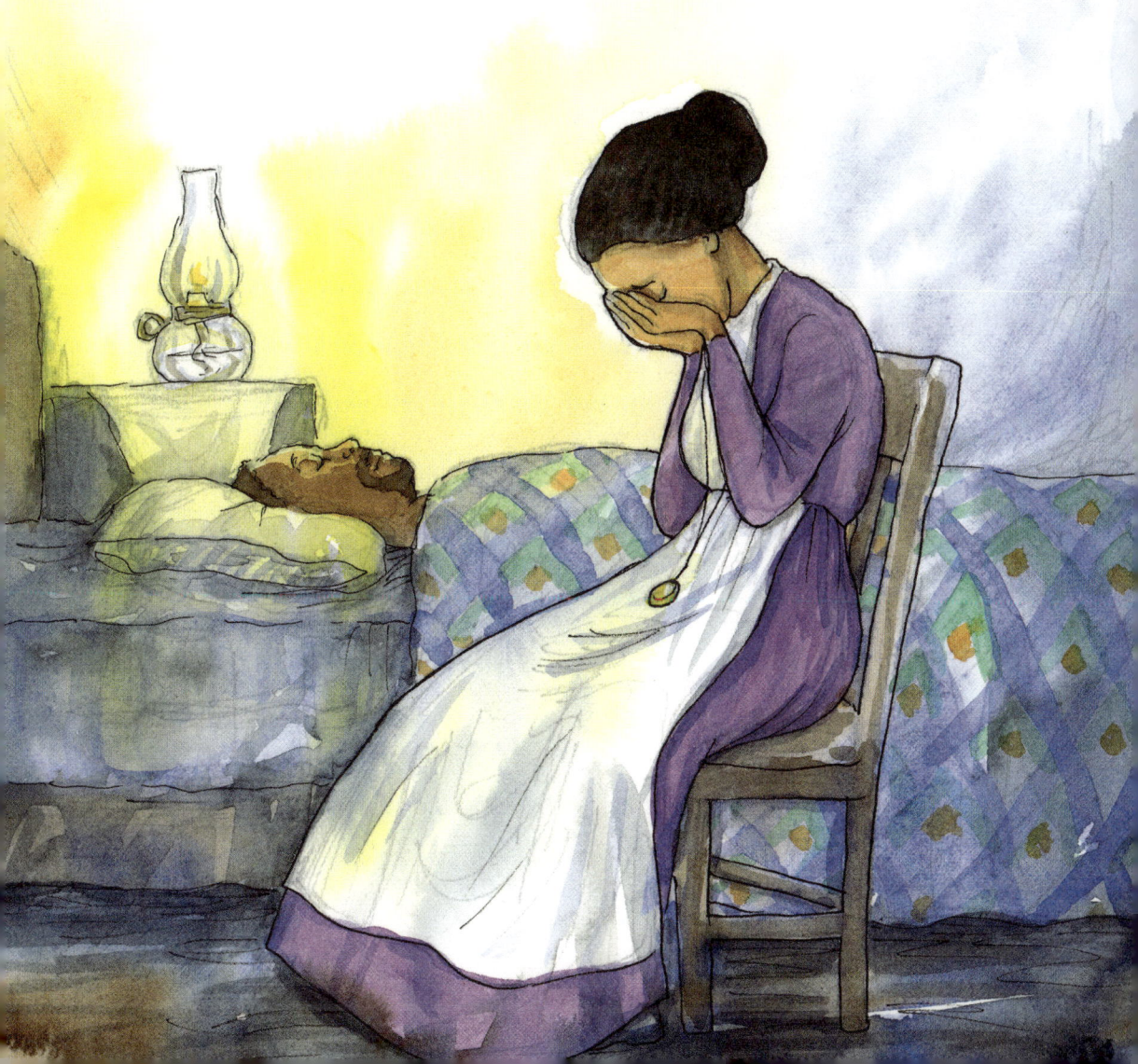

When she returned to the college after Wyatt's death, the school had cancelled her scholarship, possibly due to its financial troubles at the time. Determined as always, Rebecca applied for the new Wade Scholarship Fund, which was funded by abolitionist John Wade to support women who couldn't pay for medical education. She received an award and resumed her education.

Rebecca graduated from the medical school in 1864. It is unclear whether she knew that she was the first Black woman in America to receive a medical degree. In 1860, only about 300 of the 54,543 physicians in the United States were women, and none of those women were Black.

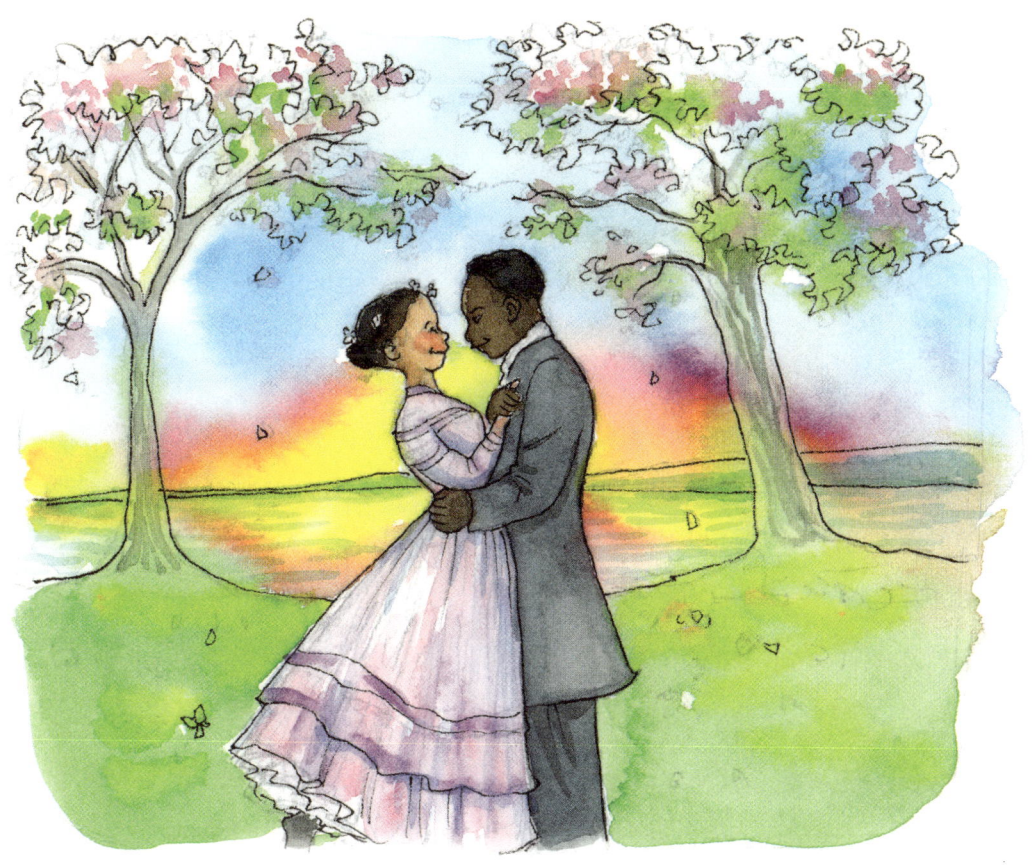

In 1865, Rebecca married Arthur Crumpler, who had escaped slavery and made his way north to freedom. Arriving in Boston in 1862, he had been sheltered by abolitionists and is thought to have been taken in by Nathaniel Allen, among others. Quite possibly it was Nathaniel who introduced Arthur to Rebecca. They were married in St. John, New Brunswick.

At the beginning of April 1865, Richmond, Virginia, the capital city of the Confederacy, fell to Union forces. Confederate General Robert E. Lee surrendered to Union General Ulysses S. Grant a week later, and the Civil War finally ended.

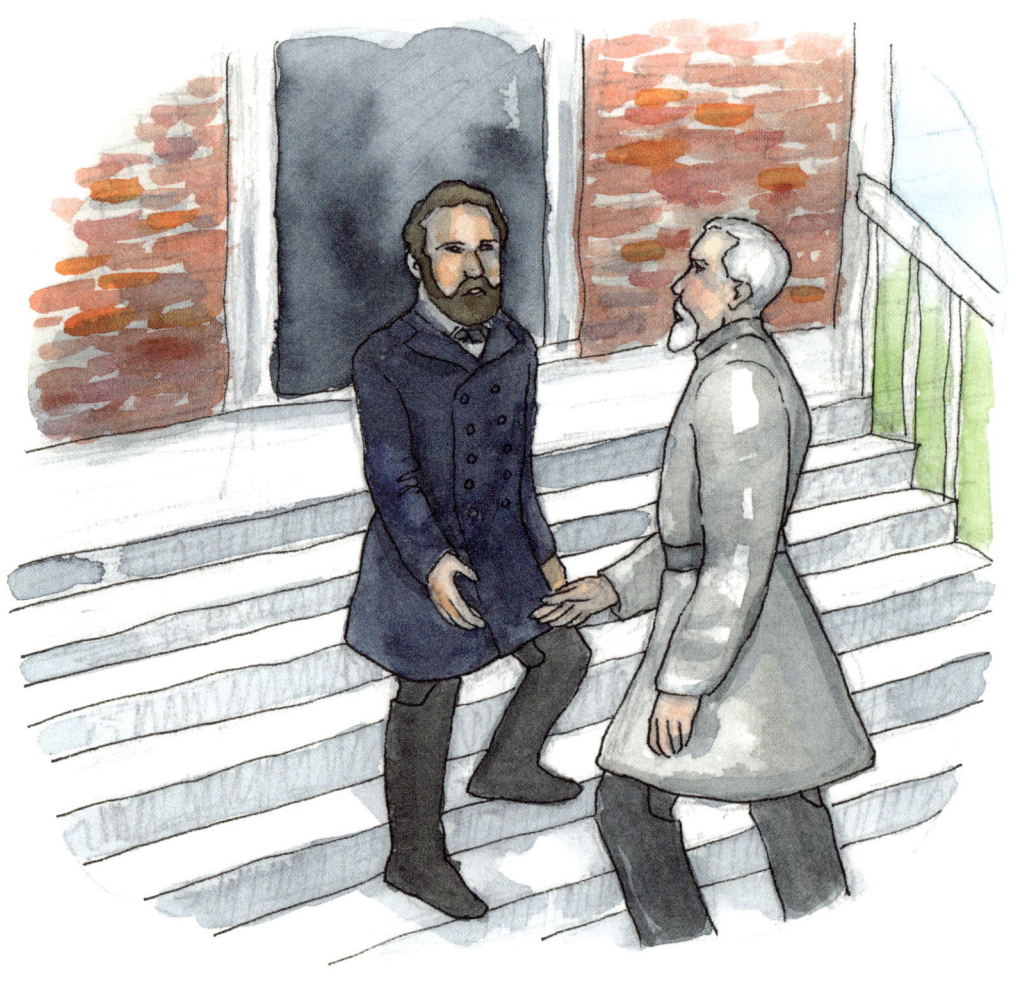

Shortly after, with Arthur at her side, Rebecca traveled to the devastated city of Richmond to work with the Freedmen's Bureau, an organization that provided food, shelter, and medical care to formerly enslaved people in an effort to help them transition to freedom.

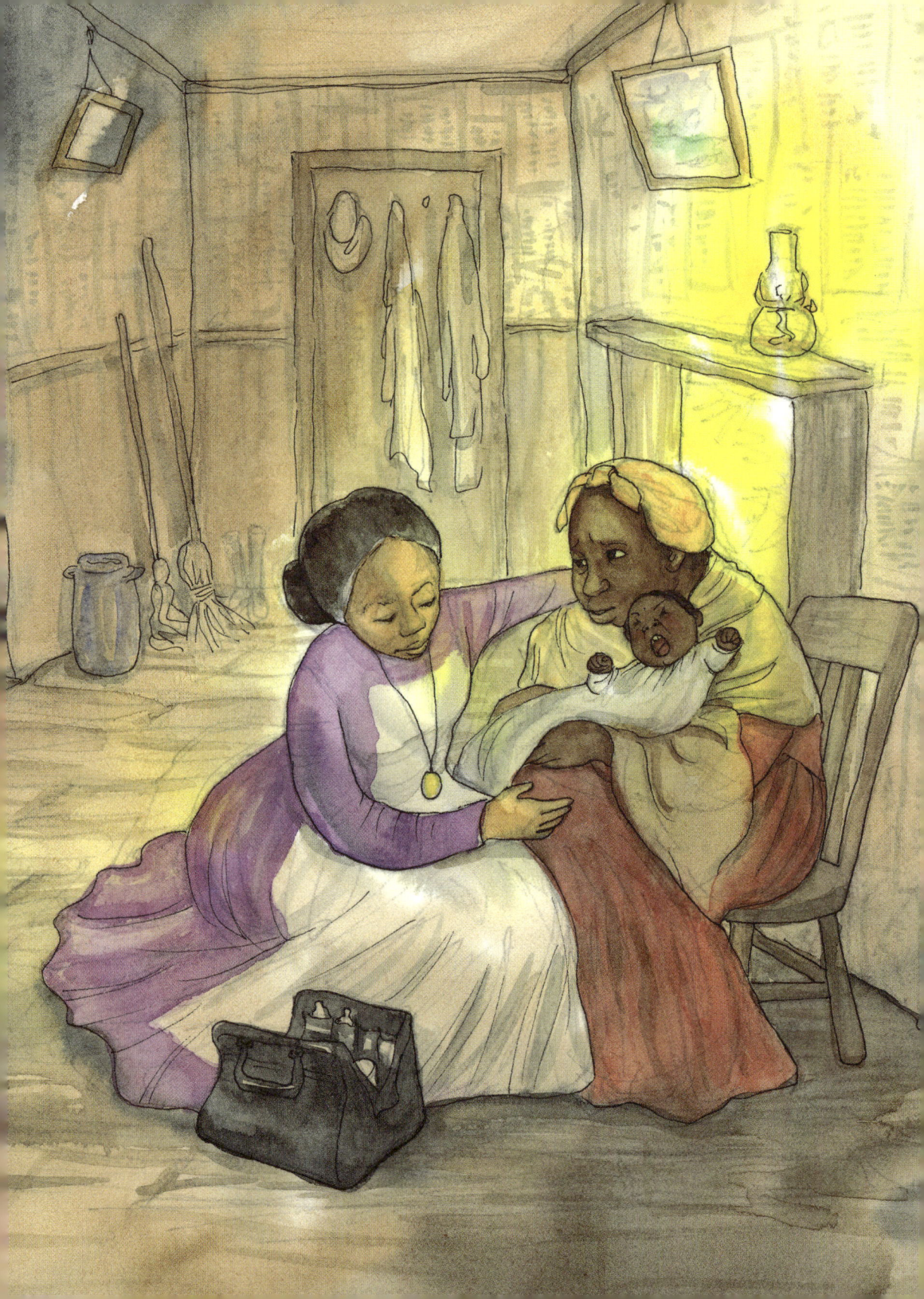

Rebecca was promoted quickly and worked in a community of over 30,000 African American men, women, and children. In her book she wrote the experience gave her "ample opportunities to become acquainted with the diseases of women and children."

She worked in Richmond's Black community for four years. While there, Arthur searched unsuccessfully for his family members, who had been separated from one another by their sale as slaves years before.

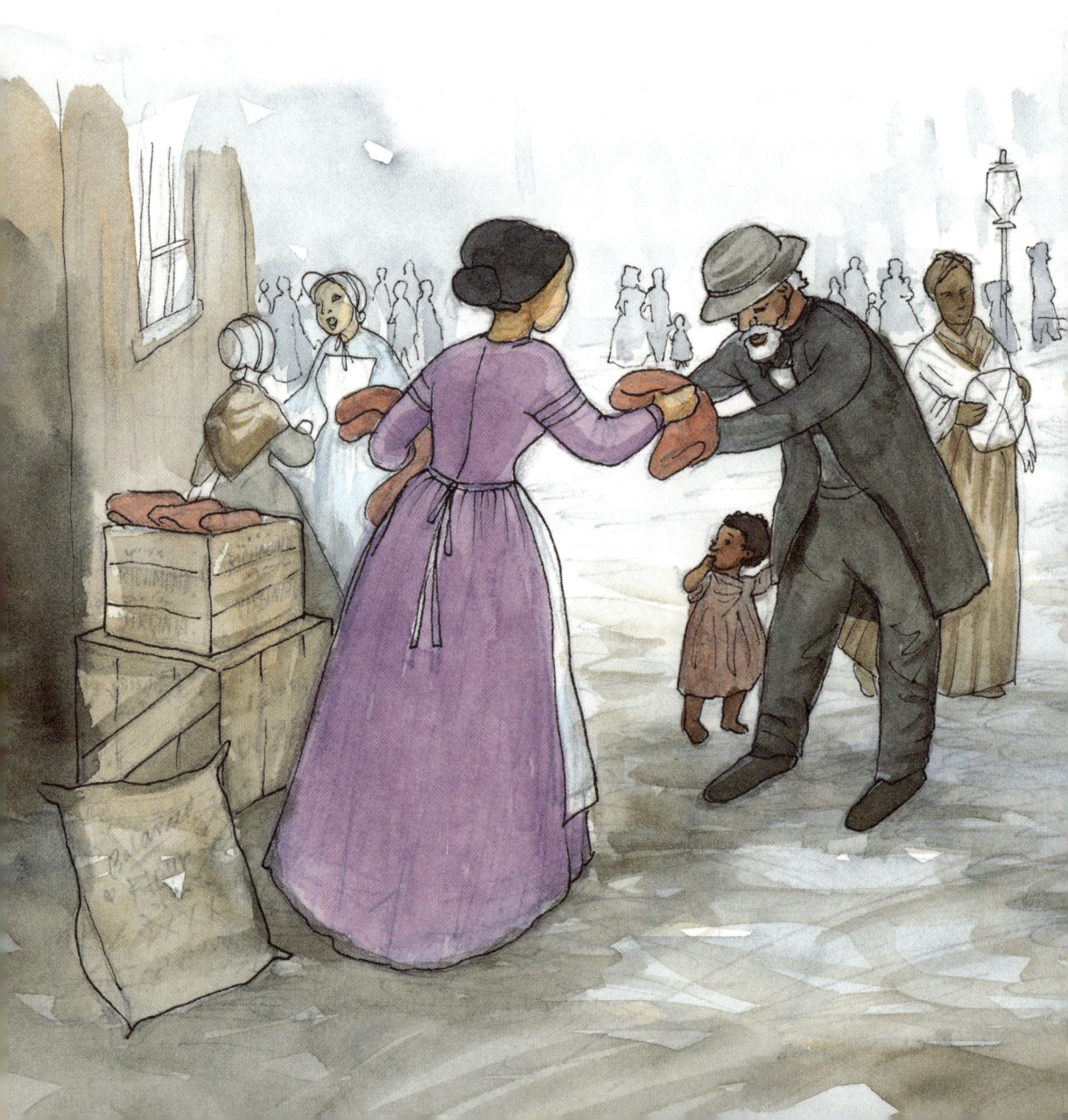

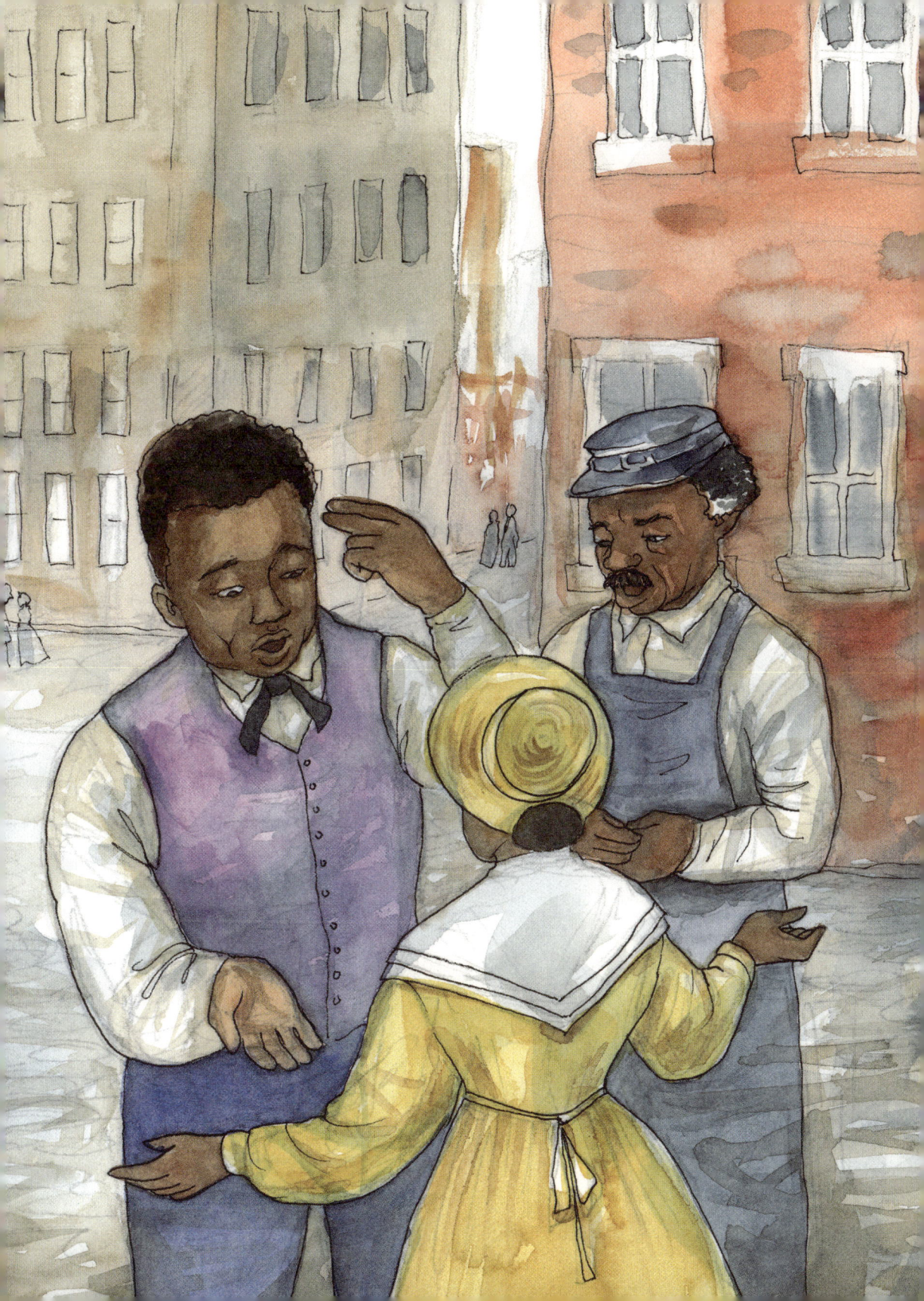

In 1869, Rebecca and Arthur returned to Boston and took up residence at 67 Joy Street, in a community on the north slope of Beacon Hill, a neighborhood of Black residents. There, she provided free care to those who needed it. Midwifery and pediatric care were desperately needed in the growing city, providing Rebecca with a nonstop stream of patients. Her reputation grew. In 1870, she gave birth to her own daughter, Lizzie Crumpler.

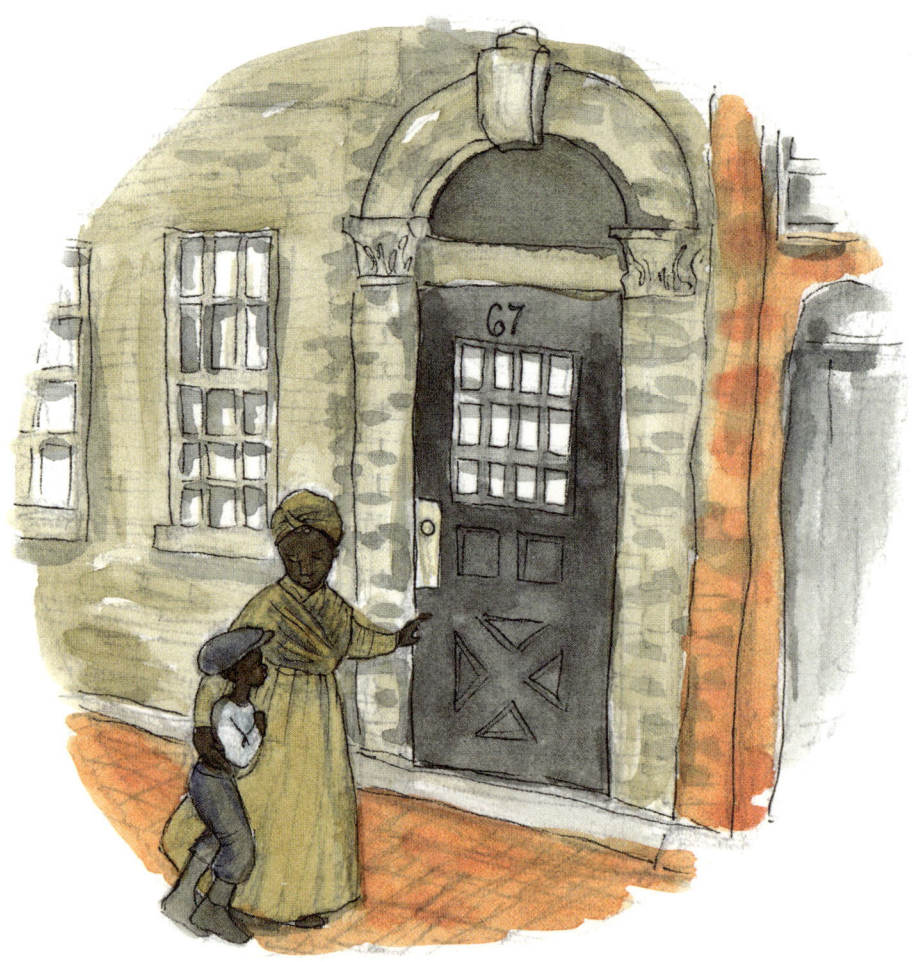

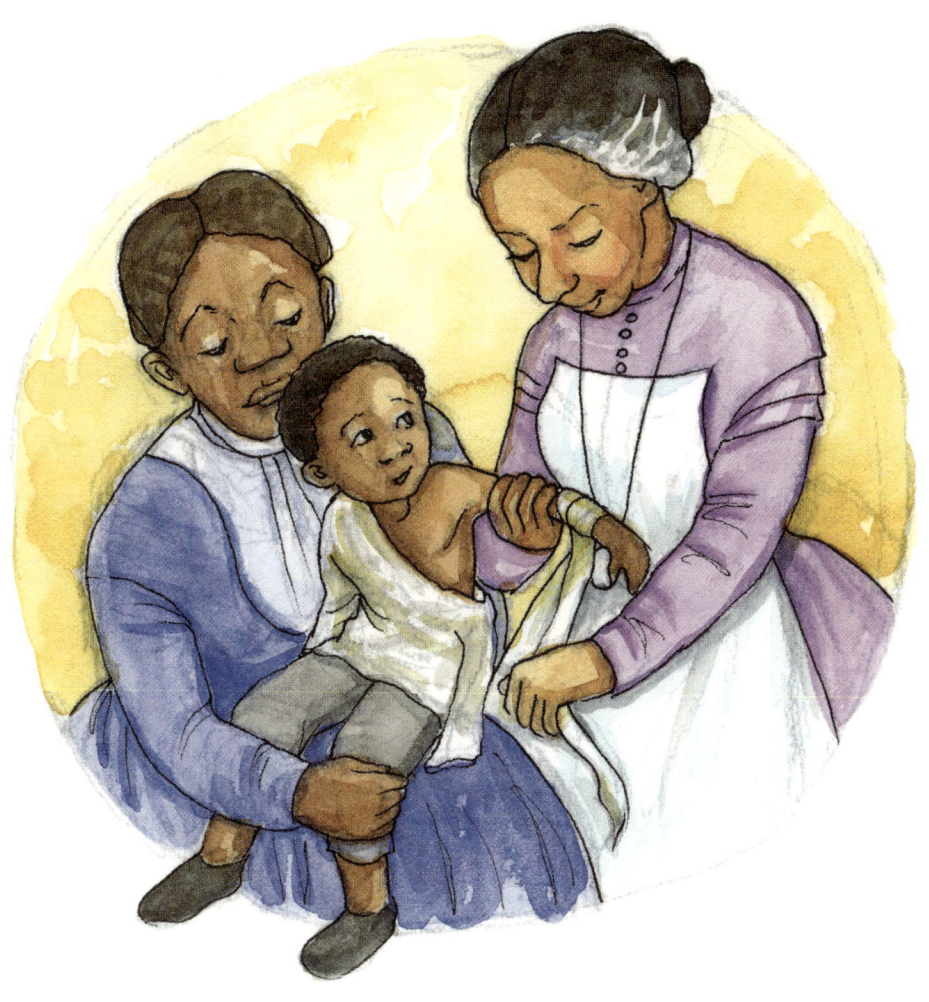

"[I was] practicing outside and receiving
children in the house for treatment;
regardless, in measure, of remuneration."

—DR. REBECCA LEE CRUMPLER

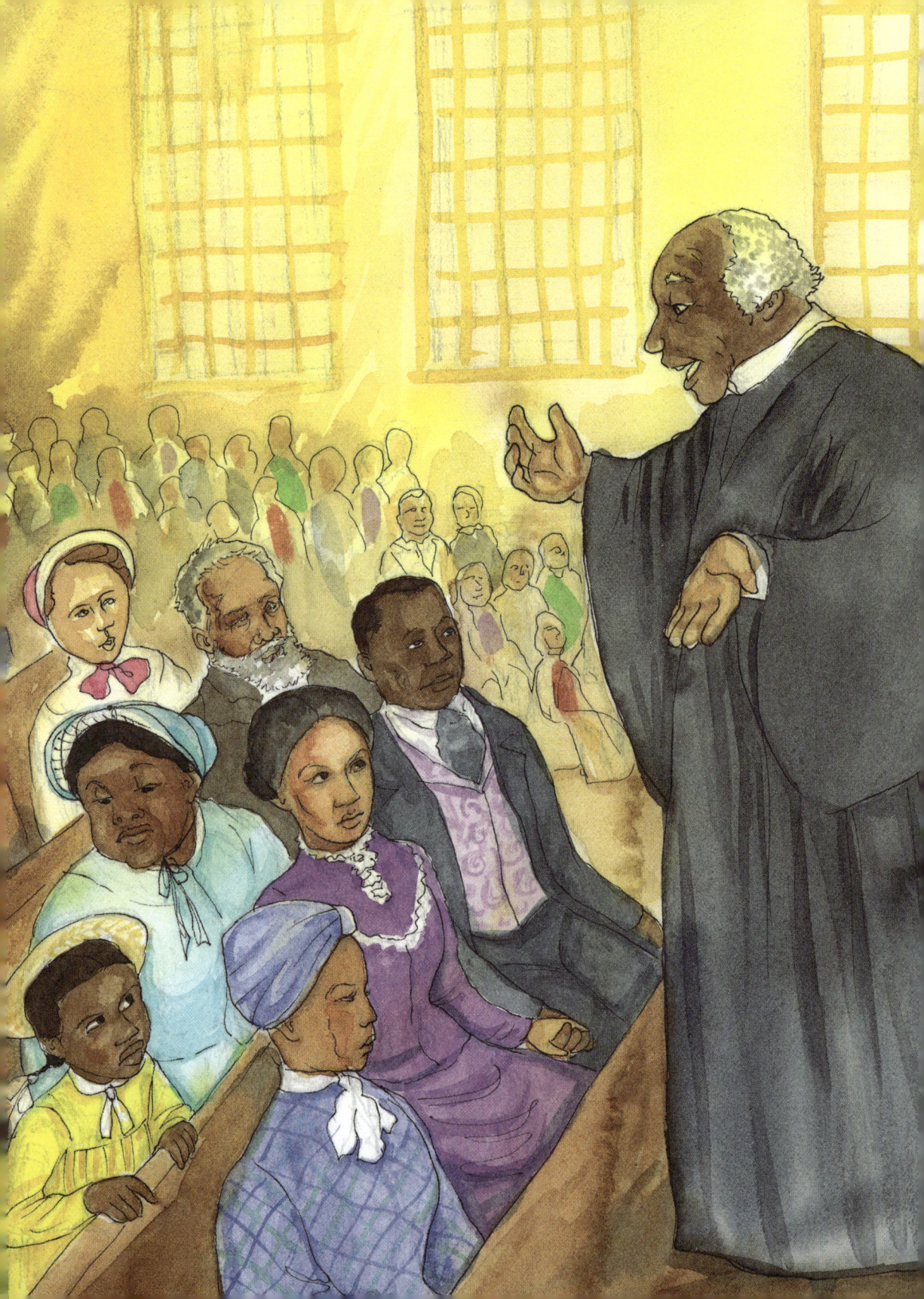

Rebecca and Arthur began attending the Twelfth Baptist Church, which was known for its high-powered, wealthy, influential Black members. The church was a frequent meeting place for abolitionists, suffragists, and activists. Its early membership rolls included many prominent Beacon Hill abolitionists.

The church had been a stop on the Underground Railroad prior to emancipation and continued to advocate for Black civil rights after the war. This advocacy was still ongoing when a young Boston University student named Martin Luther King, Jr. attended the church in the 1950s, and it continues today.

After retiring from her practice in the 1870s, Rebecca taught at her old West Newton school. She also returned to Wilmington, Delaware, to teach. Sometime between 1876 and 1880, Rebecca, Arthur, and Lizzie moved to Hyde Park, a southern suburb of Boston. There she wrote *Medical Discourses*, which a Boston-area publisher brought out in 1883.

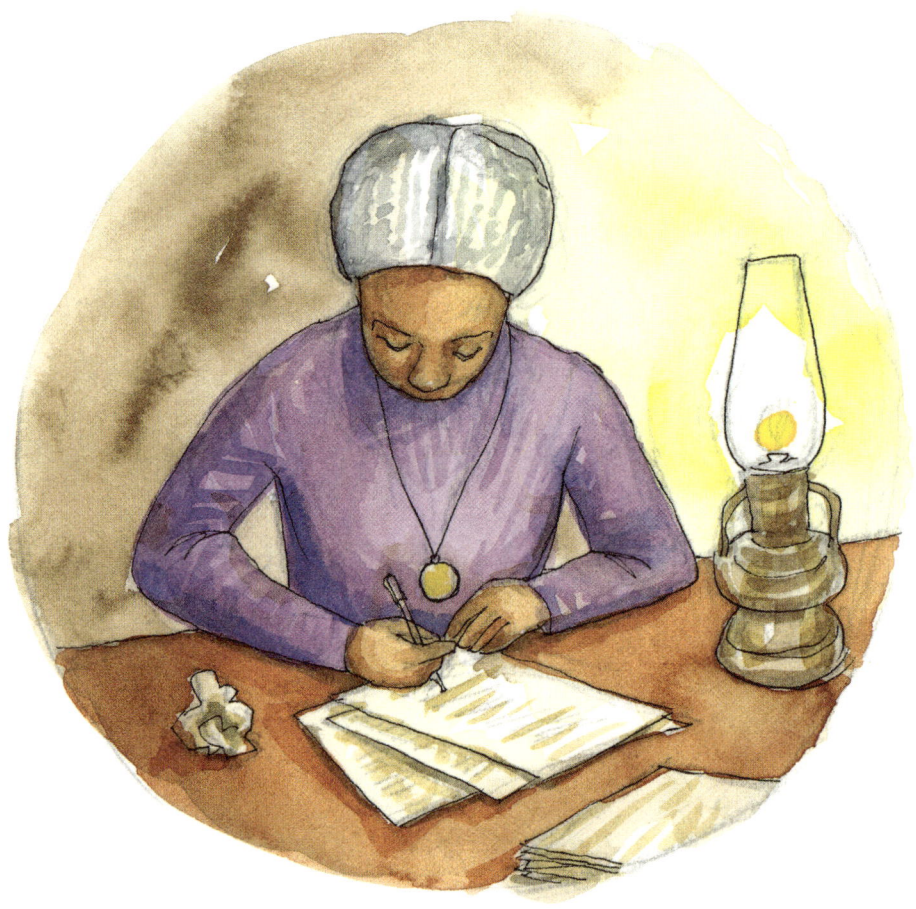

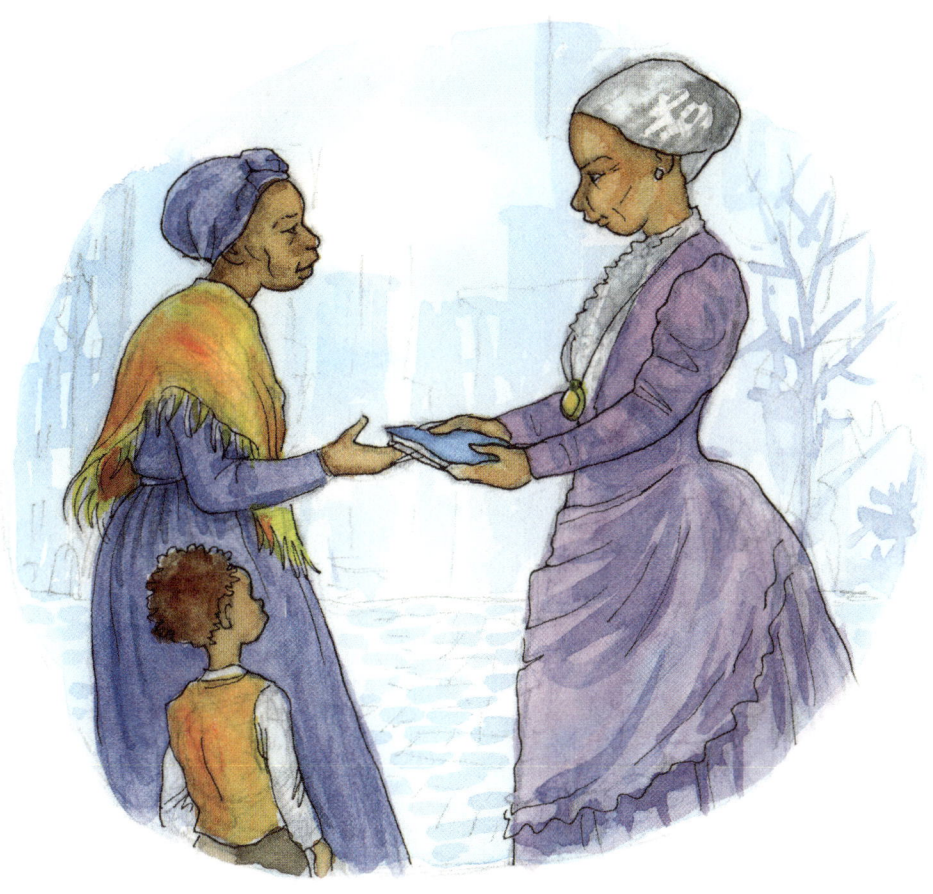

Medical Discourses made Rebecca the first Black woman physician to publish a book. It advised women on matters of maternal and pediatric health and had clear descriptions of common diseases and their early warning signs. It offered practical advice for checking and treating symptoms. It emphasized hygiene and refuted false rumors that jeopardized health.

With knowledge gained by her experiences caring for postwar communities in Virginia, Rebecca paid close attention to environmental factors that contribute to health. Now doctors call these factors "social determinants of health"—things like housing, education, healthy food, and safe relationships.

In *Medical Discourses*, Rebecca begged women to aspire to medical careers in spite of the challenges. Women can make excellent medical providers, she told her readers.

"What we need today in every community, is, not a shrinking or flagging of womanly usefulness in this field of labor, but renewed and courageous readiness to do when and wherever duty calls."

—DR. REBECCA LEE CRUMPLER

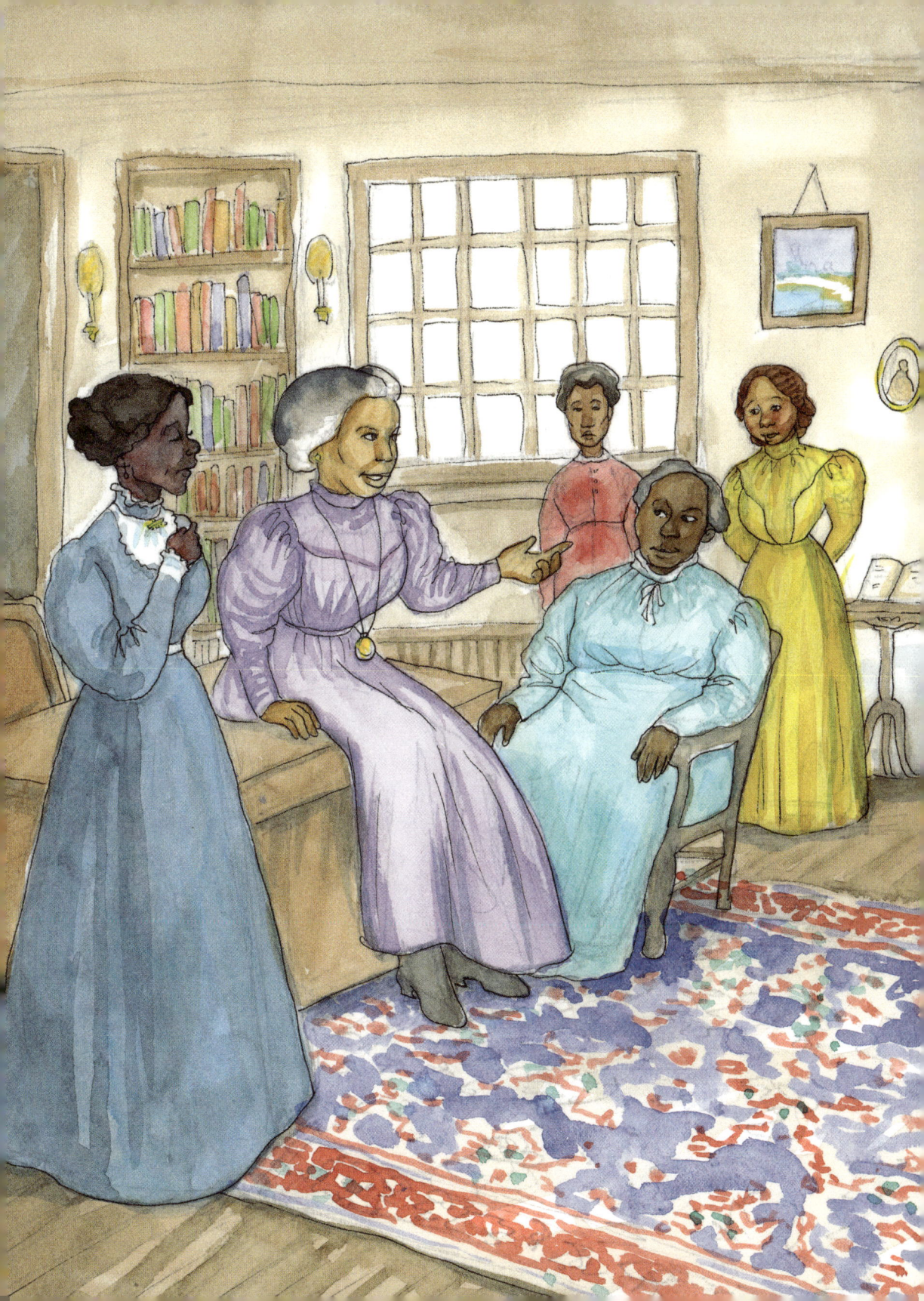

Twelve years later, at the age of 64, Rebecca died and was buried in Hyde Park's newly opened Fairview Cemetery. Her grave, like many of the early graves at Fairview, had no headstone. After Rebecca's death, Arthur moved into a single room at 43 Piedmont Street. He died in 1910 and was buried in an unmarked grave next to Rebecca.

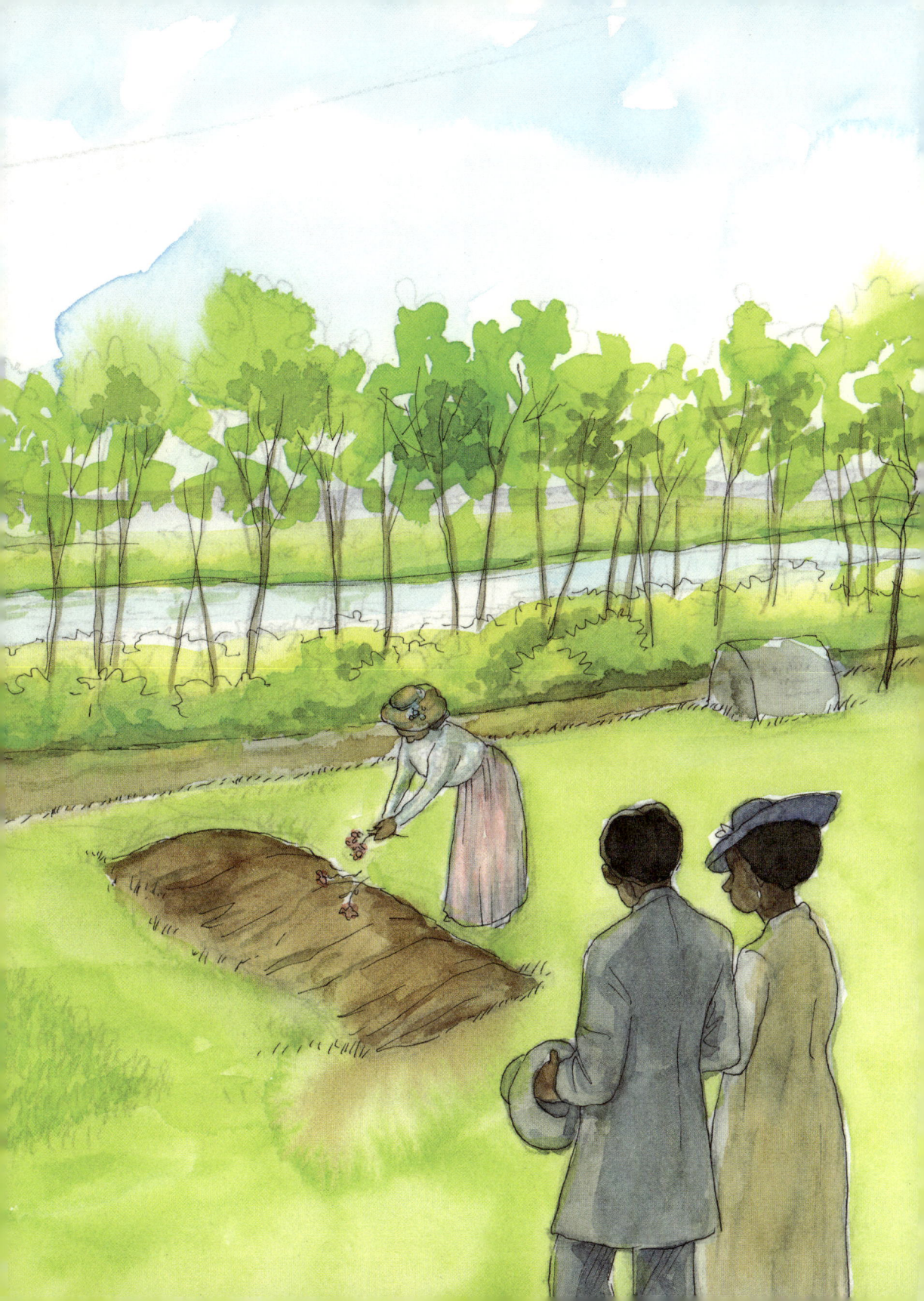

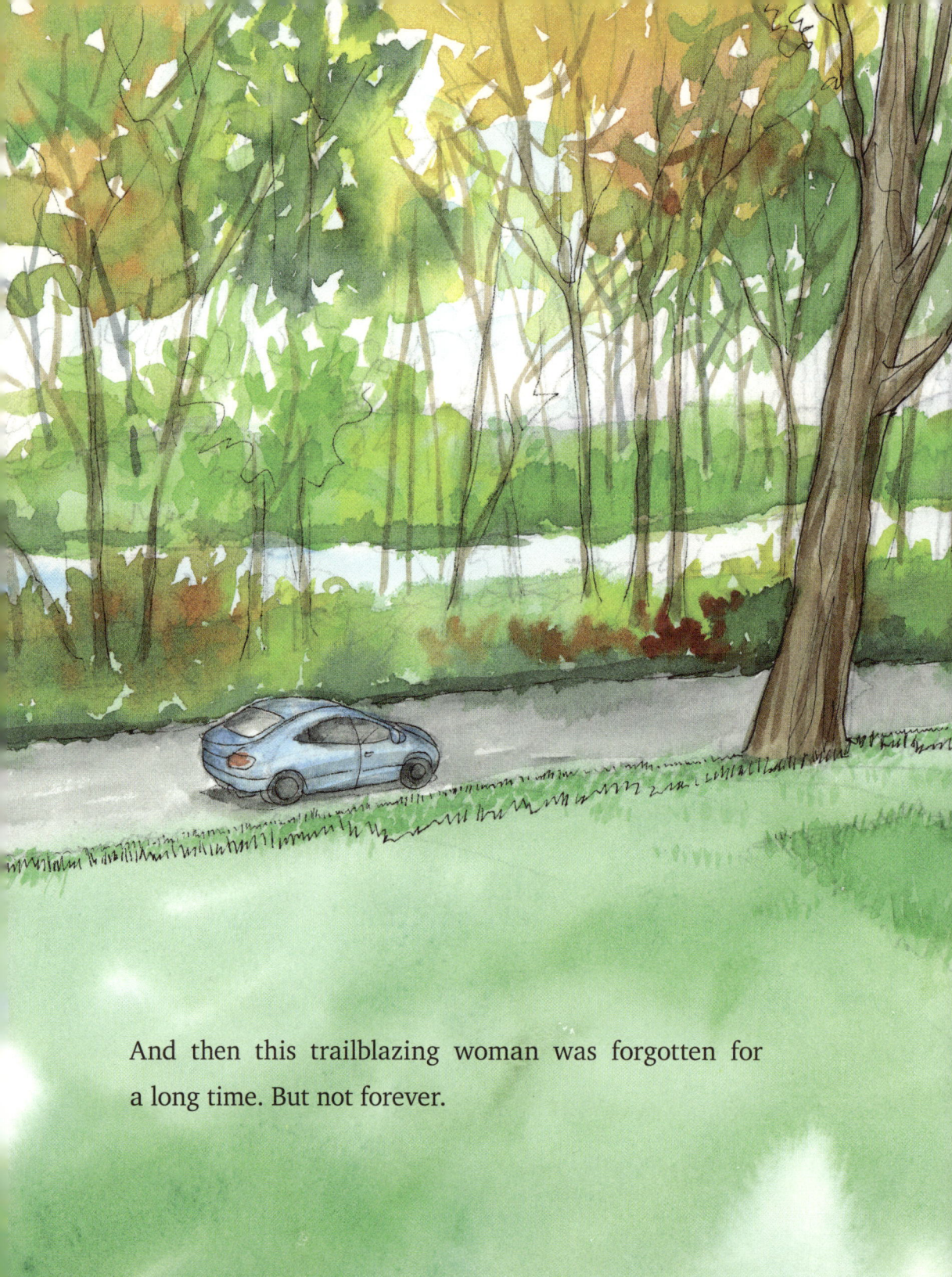

And then this trailblazing woman was forgotten for a long time. But not forever.

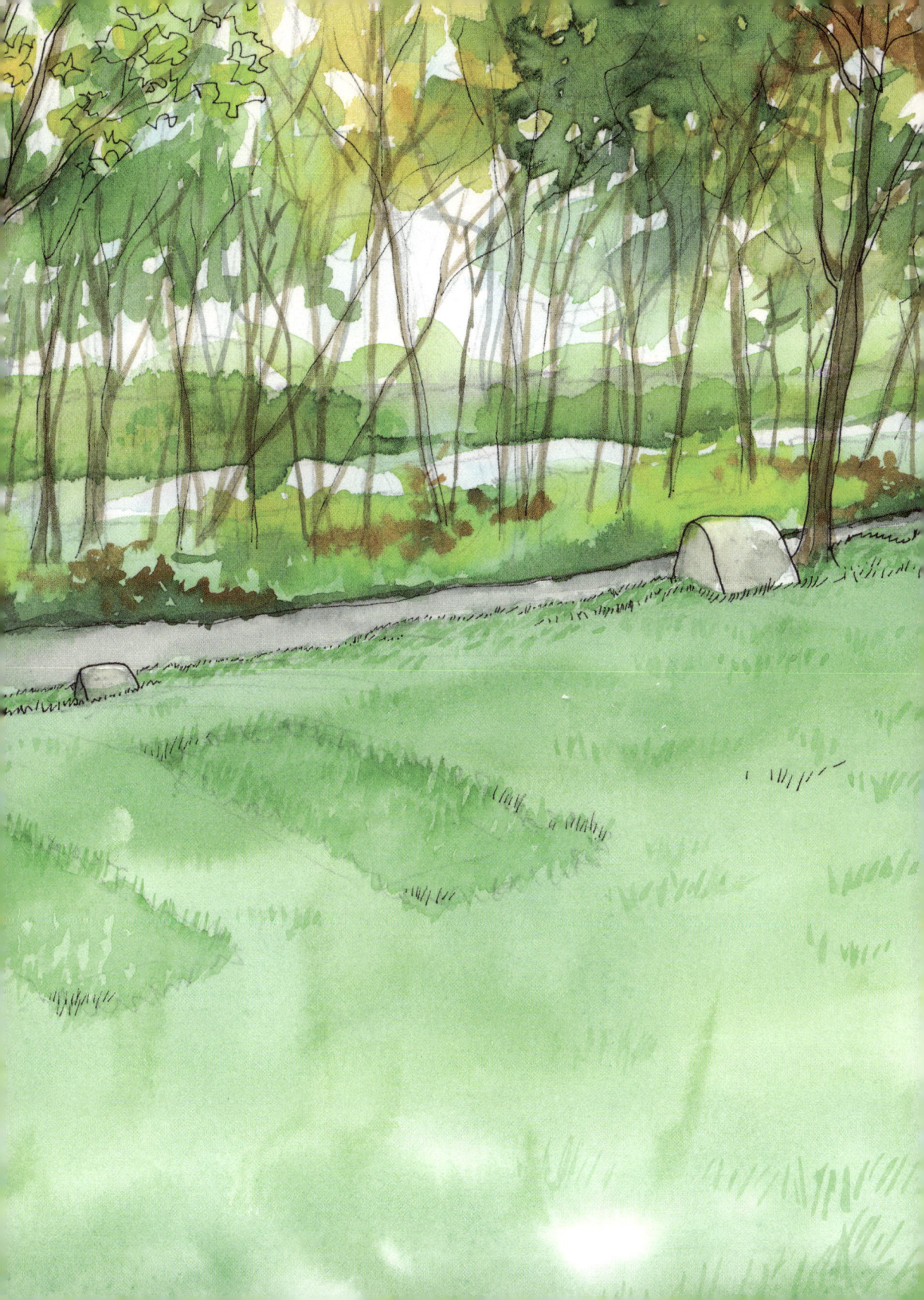

Dr. Melody T. McCloud of Rowell, Georgia, attended the Boston University School of Medicine, which had once been the New England Female Medical College, Rebecca's alma mater. Melody first learned of Rebecca through the Rebecca Lee Society, a group of Black women physicians established in the 1980s. Determined to learn more, Melody discovered all she could about Rebecca.

Rebecca's life was also researched and promoted by Dr. JudyAnn Bigby, a medical doctor, professor of medicine, and former Secretary of the Executive Office of Health and Human Services in Massachusetts. Dr. Bigby researched Black men and women in medicine throughout her career and saved articles wherever she found them, incorporating information about these pioneers into her lectures and presentations at Harvard and during visiting professorships.

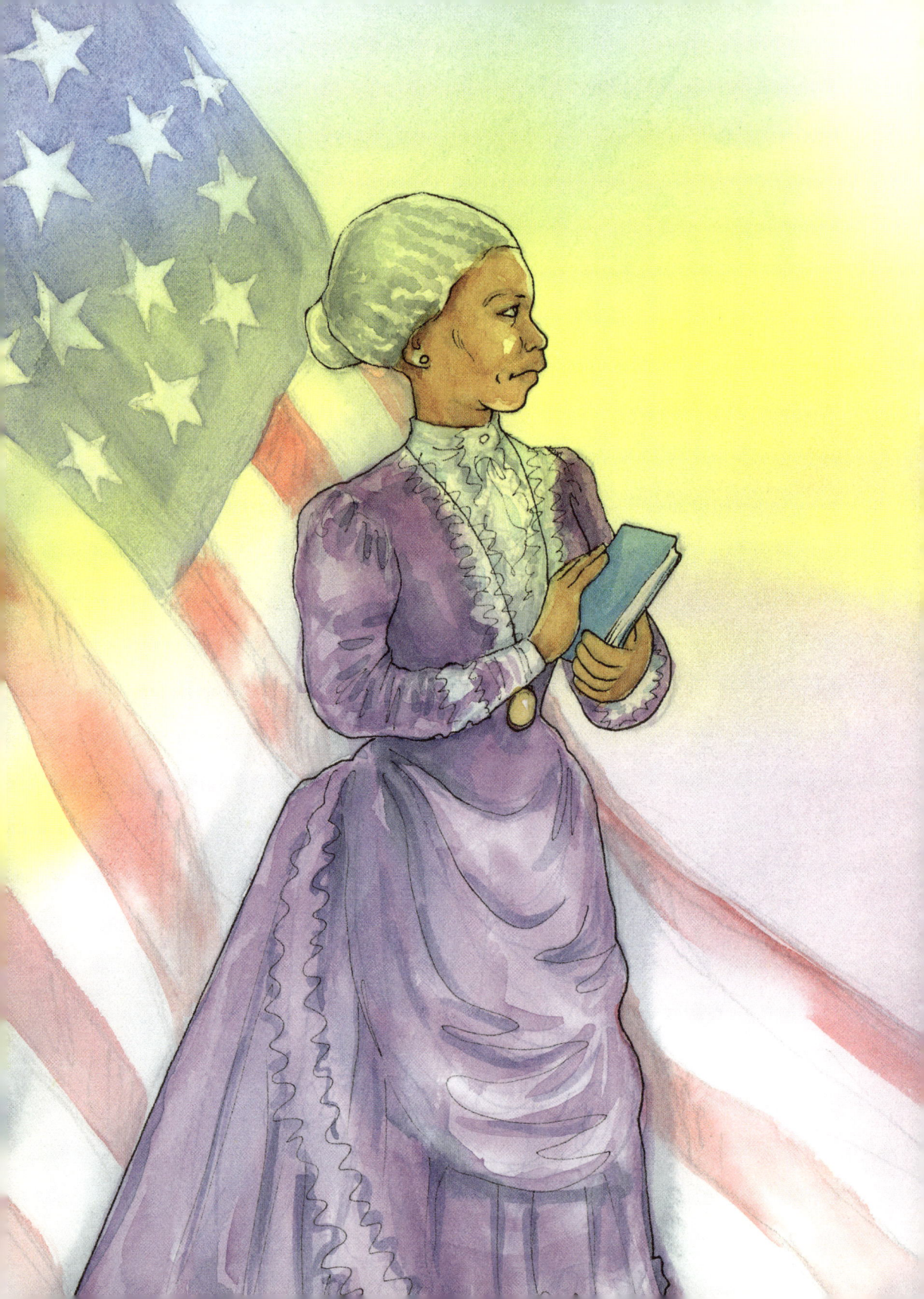

Dr. McCloud eventually succeeded in having March 30th, National Doctors Day, declared as "Dr. Rebecca Lee Crumpler Day" in Virginia, where Rebecca worked with the Freedmen's Bureau. And, after a successful fundraising campaign, Rebecca and Arthur's graves in Fairview Cemetery were adorned with proper headstones.

In 2021, the 190th anniversary of her birth, the city of Boston declared February 8th to be Dr. Rebecca Lee Crumpler Day.

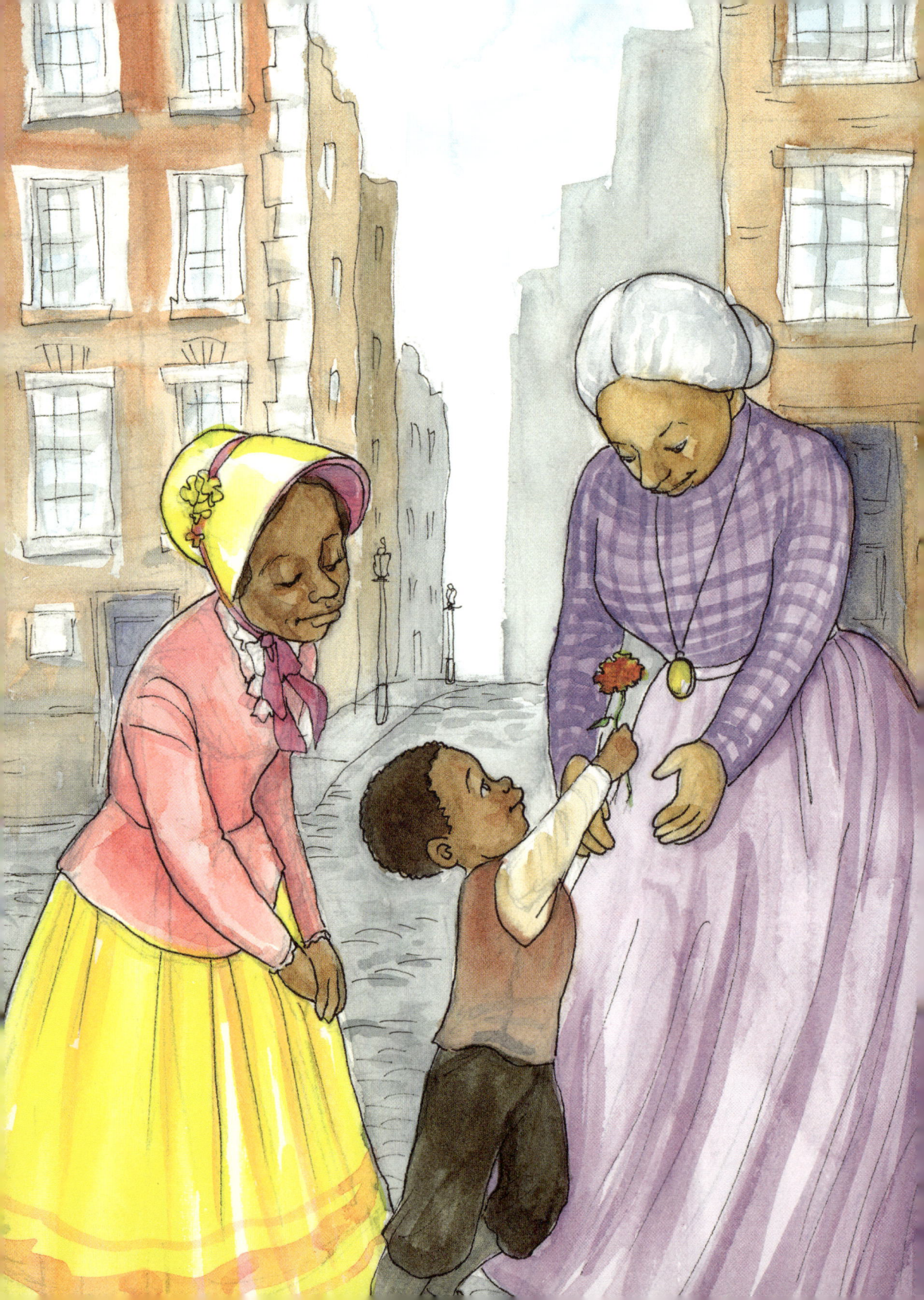

There is a lot we still don't know, but we do know that Rebecca was a trailblazer. She was brilliant. She worked hard—very hard. She was brave. She helped many people.

Rebecca Lee Crumpler,
America's first Black woman doctor.

She should be famous.
Remember her name.

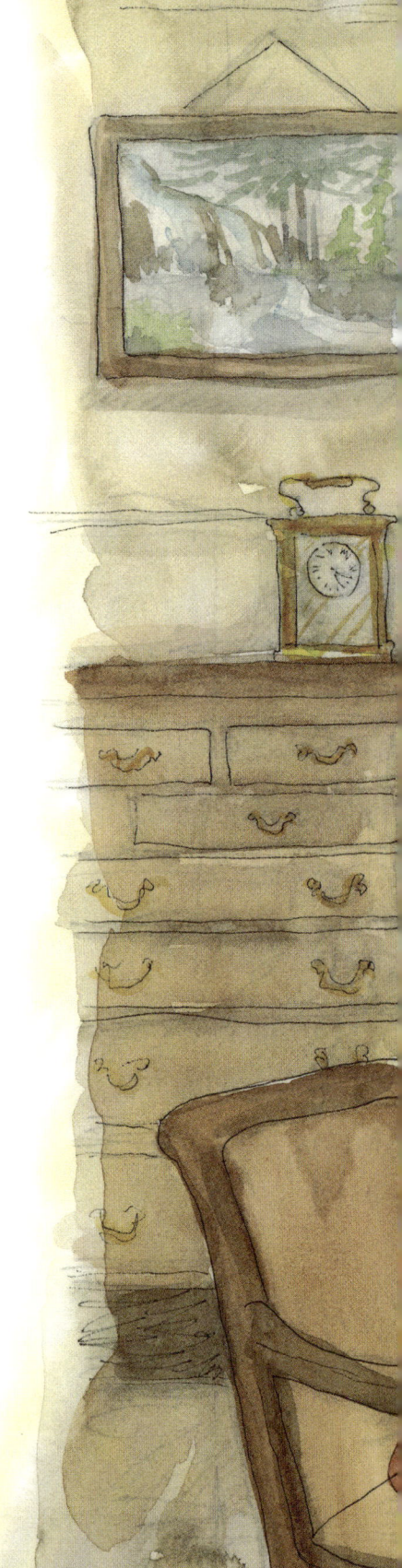

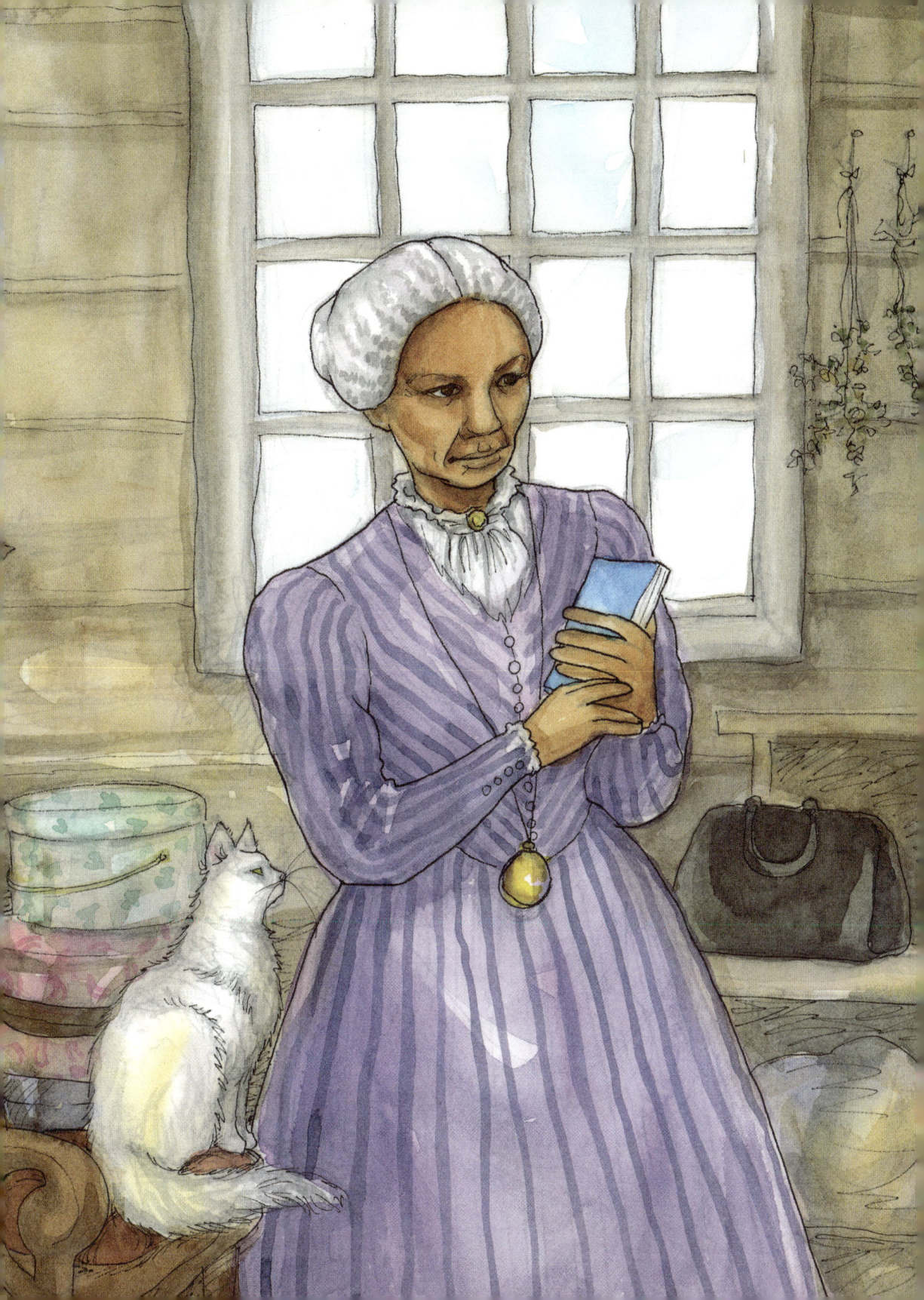

THE SEARCH FOR REBECCA

I began historical research for this project with the central primary source on Rebecca Crumpler's life—the introduction to her book, *Medical Discourses*. This is the only first-person account of her life that historians have, and it became the scaffolding onto which I built the timeline that anchored research for this project. An entry in a West Newton English and Classical School yearbook provides another important historical touchpoint, but includes an inaccuracy too. Given the dearth of concrete details, I worked to better understand the laws and conventions that governed the societies around her at the various stages of her life—early childhood in Delaware, a period in Philadelphia, medical school and licensed practice in Boston, volunteerism with the Freedmen's Bureau in Virginia, and finally, teaching in Delaware before returning to Boston—in hopes of painting a complete picture of her experience.

Some of this research was conducted online using a combination of e-books and digital archives and some was conducted in person, searching books, archives, and historical records. Poor record-keeping was common during Rebecca's life—especially during her childhood when Black families saw submitting civil records (like birth, death, and marriage certificates) as an unwelcome invitation for surveillance—and means that there are significant gaps in our knowledge.

Where family records failed, articles from local historians, reports from groups studying slavery, photographical records, and court transcripts gave further information about the experiences of Black citizens in Delaware, Boston, and Virginia. In Boston, primary sources become more accessible—marriage and address records chart Rebecca's course across the city during her early practice. Mentions of her in major newspaper articles indicate her rise to the most respected tiers of Black society. Historical books describing the histories of the medical school she attended and the neighborhoods and churches to which she devoted her time fill in additional details.

Of course, this project could not have been completed without the Dr. JudyAnn Bigbys, Dr. Melody T. McClouds, and Victoria Galls of the world—who have a passion and dedication to uncovering the truth about those who should be more famous than they are. Thank you.

SEARCHING THE ARCHIVES

Being an archivist is an important job. Archives keep and organize historical documents from the past like letters, maps, and photographs. Part of an archivist's job is to preserve, or save, these materials so that people can use them for research in the future. We use archival documents to help uncover stories of people from the past. Sometimes, it can be difficult to find information about someone in the archives because very little paper evidence about their lives exists. Black women, especially, often don't have much material about their lives saved in archives because, in the past, white authority figures deemed them less important. Although that can make it difficult to research Black women, we can use the little material we do have to make their stories come to life. Because there is so little evidence about their lives, it makes every document we have even more important.

UNCOVERING THE PAST

Think of your own community. Is there a mystery lost to history there waiting to be solved? Maybe a person waiting to be discovered and celebrated again? Who was the first female doctor in your town? The first Black teacher? Who designed the library or town hall building?

Pick a subject and see how much you can learn about the person by conducting research online, at the library, and through interviews with family, friends, or colleagues.

See if you can build a timeline of the person's life or get an idea of what they may have been like.

Write a journal from their perspective or a news article that celebrates their accomplishments.

And have fun! You too are a historian, you too are an author, and you too can help teach all of us about people who should be more famous than they are.

To my children, Soraya
and Matias, for whom I live.
—Shani

With love and gratitude to
Dr. George M. Yancey.
—Nicole

ABOUT THE AUTHOR

Shani Mahiri King is Vice Dean, Martha L. Minow Scholar, and a Professor of Law at Rutgers Law School. Shani is the father of two, for whom he wrote the children's books *Have I Ever Told You?* and *Have I Ever Told You Black Lives Matter?* He lives with his amazing wife, two wonderful kids, two untrained dogs, and two lovable cats in New Jersey.

ABOUT THE ILLUSTRATOR

Nicole Tadgell is an award-winning watercolor artist whose work spans more than thirty picture books for children. Born in Detroit, Michigan, Nicole was a shy child whose family moved frequently and art was an escape for her—especially in new schools where she was the only Black kid in class. Today, Nicole continues to bring stories to life while advocating for diversity in children's literature. In addition to her artwork, she visits schools and conducts lectures and workshops—and finds beauty, strength and solace in the practice of tai chi. Nicole lives in Chesapeake, Virginia.